The Psychobiology of Affective Disorders

Pfizer Symposium on Depression, Boca Raton, Florida, February 28–29, 1980

The Psychobiology of Affective Disorders

Edited by

Joseph Mendels, M.D.
Medical Director, The Fairmount Institute; Professor of Psychiatry,
University of Pennsylvania, Philadelphia, Pennsylvania

Jay D. Amsterdam, M.D.
Assistant Professor of Psychiatry, University of Pennsylvania, Philadelphia, Pennsylvania

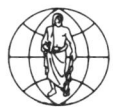

S. Karger • Basel • München • Paris • London • New York • Sydney

Although the physicians who participated in this symposium have mentioned dosages, precautions, and contraindications of drugs, the practicing physician is strongly urged to review the product information contained in the package insert of each drug before using or prescribing. For Sinequan (doxepin) prescribing information, including contraindications and adverse reactions, please see back cover.

National Library of Medicine, Cataloging in Publication
    Pfizer Symposium on Depression, Miami, Fla., 1980
    The psychobiology of affective disorders
    Editors, Joseph Mendels, Jay D. Amsterdam.–Basel; New York: Karger, 1980
    1. Depression–congresses   I. Amsterdam, Jay D., ed.   II. Mendels, Joseph, ed.   III. Title
    WM 171 P529p 1980
    ISBN 3-8055-1400-X

All rights reserved.
No part of this publication may be translated into other languages, reproduced or utilized in any form or by any means, electronic or mechanical, including photocopying, recording, microcopying, or by any information storage and retrieval system, without permission in writing from the publisher.

© Copyright 1980 by Pfizer Pharmaceuticals, New York, N.Y.
Printed in U.S.A.
ISBN 3-8055-1400-X

Contents

List of Contributors VI
Foreword VII
Acknowledgment VIII

Katz, M.M. (Washington, D.C.): Depression: A National Health Problem 1
Dunner, D.L. (Seattle, Wash.): Unipolar and Bipolar Depression: Recent Findings from
    Clinical and Biologic Studies 11
Gershon, E.S. (Bethesda, Md.): Genetic Factors from a Clinical Perspective 25
Mass, J.W. and Huang, Y. (New Haven, Conn.): Norepinephrine Neuronal System Functioning and Depression 40
Amsterdam, J.D. and Mendels, J. (Philadelphia, Pa.): Serotonergic Function and Depression 57
Frazer, A. and Mendels, J. (Philadelphia, Pa.): Effects of Antidepressant Drugs on Adrenergic Responsiveness and Receptors 72
Janowsky, D.S.; Risch, C.; Huey, L.; Parker, D.; Davis, J., and Judd, L. (San Diego, Calif.):
    The Cholinergic Nervous System and Depression 83
Carroll, B.J. (Ann Arbor, Mich.): Neuroendocrine Aspects of Depression: Theoretical and
    Practical Significance 99
Hartman, B.K.; Preskorn, S.H.; Raichle, M.E.; Swanson, L.W., and Clark, H.B. (St.
    Louis, Mo.): Effect of Tricyclic Antidepressants on Cerebral Capillary Permeability:
    An Action on a Fundamental Cerebral Homeostatic Mechanism 111
Secunda, S.K. (Bethesda, Md.): Doxepin: Recent Pharmacologic and Clinical Studies 130
Hawkins, D.R. (Chicago, Ill.): Sleep and Circadian Rhythm Disturbances in Depression . . 147
Winokur, G. (Iowa City, Iowa): Translation of Psychiatric Research into Clinical Practice . 166
Lipton, M.A. (Chapel Hill, N.C.): New Vistas: Depression Research Excluding Norepinephrine, Serotonin, Neuroendocrinology, Cholinergic Systems, and Genetics 177
Amsterdam, J.D. and Mendels, J. (Philadelphia, Pa.): Summary of New Research Strategies
    in Affective Illness 201

Author Index 209
Subject Index 211

List of Contributors

Jay D. Amsterdam, M.D., Assistant Professor of Psychiatry, University of Pennsylvania, Philadelphia, Pennsylvania

Bernard J. Carroll, M.D., Ph.D., Director, Clinical Studies Unit; Associate Director, Mental Health Research Institute, University of Michigan, Ann Arbor, Michigan

David L. Dunner, M.D., Chief of Psychiatry, Harborview Medical Center; Professor, Department of Psychiatry and Behavioral Sciences, University of Washington, Seattle, Washington

Alan Frazer, Ph.D., Associate Professor of Pharmacology in Psychiatry, Veterans Administration Hospital and Departments of Psychiatry and Pharmacology, University of Pennsylvania School of Medicine, Philadelphia, Pennsylvania

Elliot S. Gershon, M.D., Chief, Section on Psychogenetics, Biological Psychiatry Branch, National Institute of Mental Health, Bethesda, Maryland

Boyd K. Hartman, M.D., Professor of Psychiatry, Associate Professor of Neurobiology, Washington University School of Medicine, St. Louis, Missouri

David R. Hawkins, M.D., Director, Consultation-Liaison Service, Department of Psychiatry, Michael Reese Medical Center; Professor of Psychiatry, Pritzker School of Medicine, University of Chicago, Chicago, Illinois

David S. Janowsky, M.D., Director, Mental Health Clinical Research Center, Veterans Administration Medical Center, San Diego, California; Professor of Psychiatry, University of California at San Diego

Martin M. Katz, Ph.D., Clinical Professor, Department of Psychiatry and Behavioral Sciences, George Washington University Medical Center, Washington, D.C.

Morris A. Lipton, Ph.D., M.D., Sarah Graham Kenan Distinguished Professor of Psychiatry; Director, Biological Sciences Research Center, University of North Carolina School of Medicine, Chapel Hill, North Carolina

James W. Maas, M.D., Professor of Psychiatry, Department of Psychiatry, Yale University School of Medicine, New Haven, Connecticut

Joseph Mendels, M.D., Medical Director, The Fairmount Institute; Professor of Psychiatry, University of Pennsylvania, Philadelphia, Pennsylvania

Steven K. Secunda, M.D. Consultant, Clinical Research Branch, National Institute of Mental Health, Bethesda, Maryland

George Winokur, M.D., Paul W. Penningroth Professor and Head, Department of Psychiatry, University of Iowa College of Medicine, Iowa City, Iowa

Foreword

This volume records the proceedings of a symposium held on February 28–29, 1980, when a group of experts gathered to review our current knowledge of the psychobiologic factors associated with clinical depression. Attention was concentrated on those areas where data suggests that biologic factors may be important in our understanding of the etiology of depression or of its response to different forms of psychopharmacologic treatment.

Our discussions were underlined by the acknowledgment of several fundamental factors: depression is a heterogeneous illness consisting of several discrete conditions and various biologic factors may contribute to the development of some, but not all, of these illnesses; psychologic and environmental factors may also be important and may precipitate a clinical depression in their own right or by interacting with a genetic-biochemical vulnerability; the limitations of technology, and the recognition that, while research strategies have become increasingly sophisticated, there are still numerous complex biochemical variables and interactions which cannot be adequately measured in our patients; and finally, an awareness of the many homeostatic systems present in the central nervous system and the interactions which exist between these systems.

The meeting was characterized by a sense of purpose and a spirit of optimism and confidence that, in spite of many problems, we are making significant advances in this field. There was a sense that our understanding of this complex and common problem has improved significantly, and that there is great potential for an increasingly rational approach to its diagnosis and therapy.

Joseph Mendels

Acknowledgment

The papers in this volume are based on a symposium produced by Science & Medicine, Inc. and supported by a grant from Pfizer Pharmaceuticals, Inc.

Editorial assistance was provided by *Niza Leichtman-Davidson*, Ph.D.

The Psychobiology of Affective Disorders. Pfizer Symp. Depression, Boca Raton 1980, pp. 1–10 (Karger, Basel 1980)

Depression: A National Health Problem

Martin M. Katz

Department of Psychiatry and Behavioral Sciences, George Washington University Medical Center, Washington, D.C.

Several years ago, as part of a national report, NIMH staff reviewed the status of research on the depressive disorders [1]. We noted in 1973 that for the mental health professions these disorders had begun to rival schizophrenia in the sheer magnitude of the problem and in their consequent demand on services. Further, in reviewing the results of a survey on the pattern of psychotropic drug use in the USA, it turned out that upwards of 30% of the general population was reporting significant psychic distress, and that fully half of this group acknowledged symptomatology of a primarily depressive nature [2]. The 15% population figure was not an isolated statistic but apparently was replicated in at least two other similar studies [3].

In a more recent national survey, where a self-report device was used specifically designed for assessing extent of depression, 3% of the population had scores falling within the range of serious psychopathology [4]. This latter figure corresponds to the worldwide figures from epidemiologic studies which estimate the point-prevalence level between 2 and 4% [5].

There is, the reader will note, an obvious gap between the 15 and 4% figures. If we reserve the lower figure for the severe cases, or for cases which are easily identifiable clinically, then there is apparently another group, up to 10% of the population, which needs further study and possibly clinical assistance in meeting their life problems. All these figures have been under continuing surveillance by the World Health Organization, which, at one time, also identified depression as a growing and serious problem throughout the world [6]. WHO has since launched a series of studies designed to develop the means to identify depression in different cultures and to better understand its nature. I will describe those studies briefly later in this report.

Those associated with research on depression at a national level have had to try to get behind the meaning of these figures to understand their full implications for current research and treatment efforts, and to determine what they portend for the future. To approach this issue, we must ask (1) why is the incidence of depression increasing; (2) are our current methods sufficiently sensitive and valid for identifying it, for measuring its severity, and for classifying it into clinical subtypes; and (3) are our methods of treating the various depressive disorders effective?

Why Is the Incidence of Depression Increasing?

Actually, the incidence of depression may *not* really be increasing. It is possible that the professions have simply, for various reasons, increased their sensitivity, or begun to utilize methods not available in the past for its detection which make it appear more prevalent. The discovery in the early '60s of drugs for the treatment of affective disorders may also have increased our motivation to find and label certain types of disorders as depression. Such disorders were not called depression before the availability of effective treatments. It is not the first time that this has happened in medicine. Most investigators would agree, e.g., that there is no evidence that the extent of mania has significantly increased in the world. Yet proportionately more mania is diagnosed now than 10–20 years ago. We attribute that increase in diagnosed cases to the discovery of lithium, an effective, specific treatment for that condition (the availability of lithium apparently raised the awareness of clinicians to manic-like symptoms in patients suffering from a range of disorders). The epidemiology of depression presents, however, a different story. Even if we have not yet been able to establish beyond doubt that it is on the increase, there are strong reasons why we can expect to see patients with depressive disorders in increasing numbers in the future.

Both the World Health Organization and the National Institute of Mental Health have been highly sensitive to certain of these reasons: (1) with the increased life expectancy observed in most countries of the world, the proportion of individuals who are at risk for developing an age-related depressive disorder increases; (2) an increase in morbidity from chronic cardiovascular diseases, cerebrovascular and other neurologic diseases has been shown to be associated with depressive reactions in as many as 20% of all cases [1]; (3) the rapidly changing psychosocial environment of man, which often gives rise to situations of acute or prolonged environmental stress, may lead to an increase in depressive reactions [6]. The WHO, for example, sees more and more people in some countries being uprooted with resultant family disintegration (e.g., the ever increasing migrant problem in Europe and Asia); and in the USA rising divorce rates are leading to increasing social isolation among young and middle-aged adults; (4) the stresses of urbanization for hitherto primarily rural populations are expected to increase psychic disorders of all types. In this context, the widely divergent epidemiologic figures from Africa are viewed as the result of actual changes in the culture over the past 30–40 years rather than as discrepancies in data. Before the mid-Fifties, almost all such studies reported depression to be rare or nonexistent in Africans. Studies after 1955 indicate that while depression may not be highly frequent, it is certainly not uncommon [7]. Contrasting figures for urban and rural studies support the likelihood that urbanization is a critical force underlying these results [8].

Yet another possible reason for the increased numbers of cases of depressive disorders is the increasing and long-term use in most societies of medications known to induce temporary, if not chronic, depressive states. These include the phenothiazines, certain antihypertensive agents, and the oral contraceptives. It is sometimes easy for us to forget that reserpine, an effective antihypertensive drug, because of its capacity to induce a condition in some normal subjects so much like depression, strongly influenced the theory about the disorder, actually contributing to the generation of the catecholamine hypothesis of the neurochemical factors underlying the clinical condition. It is strange that we have not devoted more time to studying the association between the conditions of hypertension and depression. It is unusual that more effort has not been spent on the development of antihypertensive agents without central effects on mood.

On the Identification and Diagnosis of Depression

These are the reasons why the frequency of depressive disorders will increase in the future. If that is the case, we must ask whether our current methods for detecting, identifying, and classifying such disorders are valid and sensitive.

There is an interesting history to this whole issue of the detection and the diagnosis of the affective disorders. As both a scientific and a clinical issue, diagnosis has always been a critical and controversial problem for research in psychopathology, if not always at the center of its interest. Certain events in the Fifties and early Sixties began to increase the urgency to resolve the technical problems underlying its general applicability. For public health agencies it became clear, for example, that it would not be possible to gauge the extent of such conditions as schizophrenia and the affective disorders, if it were not possible to reliably and validly diagnose these disorders within and across national settings. There was a good deal of evidence indicating discrepancies in applications of the various classification systems within all national settings. The roots of these discrepancies were not, however, apparent. Further, and even more compelling regarding the need to resolve diagnostic issues, was the fact that drug treatments had been introduced which appeared to be highly specific, first to schizophrenia and later to depression. These drugs promised a highly significant improvement in the efficacy of psychiatric treatments, generally, if more precision and more accuracy could be achieved in the practice of diagnosis. Finally, new theories of etiology, also generated during this period, implicated genetic or biochemical sources of these conditions and were eminently testable. To test these theories, however, it was essential that valid systems of diagnoses be developed.

For these and other reasons, we have witnessed increasing concern with the process and its practice [9], and the initiation of cross-national projects designed to improve the methodology, the understanding, and the operation underlying the process of classification. The United States–Great Britain project [10], as an example of this effort, was developed to uncover the basis for the wide discrepancies in the reported prevalence of schizophrenia and the affective disorders in the USA and England. This study eventually demonstrated that the differences in mental illness statistics in the two countries were mostly owing to differences in diagnostic practice and not to the small difference in actual occurrence. The outcome of such studies made clinicians generally aware of the problems underlying the unreliability of diagnosis, and resulted in the development of newer, more systematic approaches to its conduct. The Research Diagnostic Criteria (RDC) [11] has since evolved, and under the impetus of the WHO international studies [12] and the NIMH collaborative program [13], structured interview schedules, e.g., the SADS [14], have been developed. The NIMH program utilizing these improved approaches is conducting a comparative analysis of the reliability and validity of the several classification systems currently in use in the field of depression research, e.g., the primary-secondary and the bipolar-unipolar systems. These studies should move the field of research on the affective disorders onto a sounder base so that we are in a better position to assess both in clinical and in epidemiologic studies the severity and types of conditions in question. Detecting the less severe and the masked forms of depression are, however, still somewhat beyond our reach. A number of technical and substantive issues have to be resolved in this sphere.

A significant proportion of patients, for example, go to medical clinics in the USA, and elsewhere, whose main problem is not physical but emotional, and which is often a variant of a depressive disorder. They have come to be known as "masked depressions," and are frequently not detected by the general practitioner. There are, also, those patients with a diagnosed significant physical disorder who have an associated secondary depression. Furthermore, there are those who may be under drug treatment for a physical condition, such as hypertension, who have become depressed as a direct result of the treatment. All these conditions require treatment in varying degrees of intensity for a depressive condition. The treatment prescribed for each type most likely differs. How does one detect, however, the presence of such conditions?

We should be doing more research in this sphere than is currently in progress. *Secunda* et al. [1] reported on the early results of a study conducted at a group health facility and sponsored by the NIMH. This study was aimed at (1) obtaining estimates of the prevalence of mood depression and clinically diagnosable depressive illnesses in a sample of patients consulting physicians for nonpsychiatric medical care, and (2) assessing the diagnostic and treatment practices in relation to concurrent depressive illnesses within this physician-patient sample.

The Beck Depression Inventory [15] was used to screen patients followed by a psychiatric interview. Approximately 7% of a sample of 550 patients were found to be significantly depressed. Methodology for detecting clinical depression in such cases, and in the population at large, is still a problem. A number of organizations, notably the Center for Epidemiologic Studies at NIMH, has been at work on this problem for some time. They recently launched a nationwide program which will establish centers in different parts of the country capable of conducting surveys of depressive and other disorders in the general population.

The WHO initiated studies some years ago of the characteristics of depressive disorders to study comparability of their expression in four highly diverse cultures [16]. In a second phase of that research program, it has demonstrated that comparable studies of depression in general practice patients can also be conducted in these settings. The first step in that program was the testing of a common screening interview method, which was shown to be feasible and sufficiently sensitive across these diverse national settings. Thus, the incidence of depression in the medically ill in Iran, Japan, Switzerland, India and Canada can now be compared. This work is still in progress.

One of the nagging problems in all general population studies, however, is the question of cutting points. When, for example, do the temporary phases, the natural downs of everyday living, become a subject for clinical analysis and for intervention? When does normal depression become a clinical disorder? We expect that national surveys now applying a more sophisticated psychologic methodology will be more informative about that. From all we can tell, based on the little evidence that now exists on the issue, there is no easy answer. Once a mild disorder is detected, the question clinicians will have to ask the potentially ill patients are how long these downs persist, how frequently they occur, and how much of everyday social and behavioral functioning is affected.

In a community study, *Hogarty and Katz* [17, 18] compared that segment of a normal population, who were described as the most depressed in mood, with a clinical sample of depressed outpatients. We used the same method of study for both groups. We found that as to central mood, the normal subjects appeared to significant relatives who lived with them as deeply depressed based on this experiential or subjective aspect. The normal subjects and the patients differed, however, on the descriptions of their actual behavior and social performance (i.e., whether they were still working and able to conduct everyday activities). Obviously, when normalcy or illness is at issue, more than mood and more than the subjective experience of depression are involved.

We are concerned about degrees of illness and we must know more about it; not as to identifying severe depression, which can be done quite well now, but how to discriminate within the minor forms of the condition. These minor forms make up the large proportion of the depressive disorders; they describe some 75% or more of all those who suffer from this condition. We require a finer classification here because it is in this group that finding the most appropriate treatment is such a critical art and toward which the most creative effort must now be directed.

Are Methods of Treating the Various Depressive Disorders Effective?

This brings me to the last question: How is this class of patients being treated? How should they be treated in the future? We are aware that in current practice the treatment of a depressive disorder depends on its severity and, only to a small extent, on its probable etiology. Minor forms of the disorder may be treated with psychologic counseling. However, in view of the skepticism concerning the efficacy of psychotherapeutic approaches generally, the more likely treatment will be a drug. Several classes of antidepressant drugs are available. Unless there is a real threat of suicide, clinicians will attempt to find the right drug and dosage before turning to what are considered more radical approaches to treatment, such as electroconvulsive therapy (ECT). Drugs now comprise the treatment of choice in most clinical settings.

New psychotherapeutic procedures especially designed for depression have, however, been developed over the past 10–15 years, and these methods are beginning to play a large role in its treatment. Cognitive behavior [19] and interpersonal [20] psychotherapies are two such forms which have been tested in controlled clinical trials and demonstrated to be effective. For the past 2 years, the NIMH has been trying to launch a comparative study of these psychotherapies with a standard drug treatment, attempting to extend our understanding of the manner in which the various approaches can contribute to controlling these conditions.

Without exploring all the possible approaches to treatment, certain principles seem clear. Treatment for the severe forms of depression which, in most patients, require hospitalization must rely heavily on medication and other somatic therapies. Psychotherapy in the initial stage of treatment can at best play an adjunct role. The large majority of the depressive disorders are, as we noted, seen in the outpatient departments (upwards of 75%). The etiology of the large majority of these conditions remains obscure. A segment can be depressed as a function of a specific genetic or biochemical vulnerability; another segment for reasons which are basically psychologic. The etiology of depression almost always is a function of the interaction of these processes.

We have learned in other situations that regardless of cause, chemical treatments and psychologic methods can alter clinical states in favorable directions. For a large number of patients, treatments which are both effective and efficient are urgently needed. Economy may also be a highly important consideration. The drugs are likely to remain, on the one hand, as the most preferred approach since they are currently the most effective and economical treatment for the large majority of patients. On the other hand, the minor forms of the disorder are likely to have a very large psychologic component. One might ask, then, how can the drugs serve anymore than as a short-term solution? It is possible that the fields of psychiatry and psychology are being lulled by these treatments. They are effective and highly economical of professional time but may have only short-term effects. Thus, there are obvious needs for certain kinds of research: (1) We must pursue the study of the psychologic roots of these conditions as vigorously as we are currently studying potential genetic and biologic causes. (2) We must encourage the scientific examination of promising psychologic therapies, as much for understanding how they are contributing as for determining their actual efficacies. Moreover, we must find out how such treatments might be merged with the somatic approaches. (3) Clinically, we should prepare to deal promptly with the minor forms of the condition, preferably in the practitioner's office, so that they do not graduate into more chronic conditions. (4) Through training, the general practitioner and the college counselor must be made aware more quickly of the presence of depressive disorders in the physically ill and the potential mood-altering effects of the drugs used in treating a wide range of medical conditions, particularly hypertension. (5) The routine use of antidepressant drugs in these conditions must be tempered by greater attention to their undesirable long-term side effects, and the importance of avoiding the development of chronic dependence.

Psychotropic drugs have played a critical and significant role in the clinical and research fields. They have stimulated new theories and broadened our whole grasp of the nature of depression. The search for new drugs will continue. The field, however, must now move on from this new base of knowledge to complete its unfinished work in exploring the psychologic underpinning and the experiential realm of this basically human condition.

References

1 Secunda, S.K.; Katz, M.M.; Friedman, R.; Schuyler, D.: Special Report, 1973. The depressive disorders. No. 1724-00325 (US Government Printing Office, Washington 1973).
2 Mellinger, G.D.; Balter, M.B.; Mannheimer, D.I.; Cosin, I.H.; Parry, H.J.: Psychic distress, life crisis and use of psychotherapeutic medication. Archs. gen. Psychiat. *35:* 1045–1052 (1978).
3 Mellinger, G.D.; Balter, M.B.; Mannheimer, D.I.: Patterns of psychotherapeutic drug use among adults in San Francisco. Archs. gen. Psychiat. *25:* 385–394 (1971).
4 Levitt, E.E.; Lubin, B.: Depression: concepts, controversies, and some new facts (Springer, New York 1975).
5 Lehmann, H.: Epidemiology of depressive disorders; in Fieve, Depression in the 1970s (Excerpta Medica, Amsterdam 1971).
6 Sartorius, N.: Epidemiology of depression. WHO Chron. *29:* 423–427 (1975).
7 Prince, R.: The changing picture of depressive syndromes in Africa: Is it fact or diagnostic fashion? Can. J. Afr. Stud. *1:* 177–192 (1968).
8 Marsella, A.J.: Thoughts on cross-cultural studies on the epidemiology of depression. Culture, Med. Psychiat. *2:* 343–357 (1978).
9 Katz, M.M.; Cole, J.O.; Lowery, H.A.: Studies of the diagnostic process: the influence of symptom perception, past experience, and ethnic background on diagnostic decisions. Am. J. Psychiat. *125:* 937–947 (1969).
10 Cooper, J.E.; Kendall, R.E.; Gurland, B.J.; Sharpe, L.; Copeland, J.R.M.;

Simon, R.: Psychiatric diagnoses in New York and London (Oxford University Press, London 1972).
11 Spitzer, R.L.; Endicott, J.; Robins, E.: Research diagnostic criteria: rationale and reliability. Archs. gen. Psychiat. 35: 773–782 (1978).
12 World Health Organization: Report of the International Pilot Study of Schizophrenia (WHO, Geneva 1973).
13 Katz, M.M.; Secunda, S.K.; Hirschfeld, R.M.A.; Koslow, S.H.: NIMH Clinical Research Branch collaborative program on the psychobiology of depression. Archs. gen. Psychiat. 36: 765–771 (1979).
14 Endicott, J.; Spitzer, R.L.: A diagnostic interview: the schedule for affective disorders and schizophrenia. Archs. gen. Psychiat. 35: 837–844 (1978).
15 Beck, A.T.: Depression: clinical, experimental, and theoretical aspects (Hoeber, New York 1967).
16 Sartorius, N.; Davidian, H.; Ernberg, G.; et al.: International agreement on the assessment of depression (preliminary communication). 6th Wld. Congr. of Psychiatry, Honolulu 1977.
17 Hogarty, G.; Katz, M.M.: Norms of adjustment and social behavior. Archs. gen. Psychiat. 25: 470–480 (1971).
18 Katz, M.M.: The classification of depression: normal, clinical, and ethnocultural variations; in Fieve, Depression in the 1970s (Excerpta Medica, Amsterdam 1971).
19 Beck, A.T.: Cognitive therapy and the emotional disorders. (International Universities Press, New York 1976).
20 Weissman, M.M.: Prusoff, B.A.; DiMascio, A.; Neu, C.; Goklaney, M.; Klerman, G.L.: The efficacy of drugs and psychotherapy in the treatment of acute depressive episodes. Am. J. Psychiat. 136: 555–558 (1979).

Discussion

Mendels: I am bothered by your remarks which seem to equate severity of depression, i.e., severity of symptomatology, with the etiology of depression. If you are saying that more severe illnesses are likely to have genetic, biochemical or biologic causes while milder depressions have psychologic and interpersonal causes at their core (and, therefore, respond to psychotherapeutic intervention), I cannot agree. Certainly, there are mild depressions resulting from biologic factors. Equating severity with etiology means treating according to severity. In clinical practice that should not be the case.

Carroll: I also believe that severity and etiology of depression are not directly linked. Based on my clinical experience, a mild, endogenous depression is related primarily to the patient's biologic and not to a psychologic disorder.

Katz: I did not mean to imply that severity and etiology should be equated. It is just that the evidence for a biologic basis of depression comes from studies on severely ill, hospitalized patients. That's the only evidence we have. This does not exclude the possibility that the same factors also are involved in the milder forms of depression, but there is no comparable evidence for this group. The weight of clinical theory and experience would, however, suggest that psychologic factors play a significantly larger role here. I caution clinicians not to get caught up in this.

Maas: From the practical point of view, practitioners often ask which patients benefit from drug therapy and which do not. In general, most studies indicate that among patients meeting the criteria for a major depressive disorder, 75% respond (at least moderately well) to pharmacotherapy. Among patients with milder depressions, so-called neurotic depressions, only 25% respond to drug therapy. Of this 25%, some have excellent responses. What does all this mean to the practitioner? First, when dealing with a major depressive disorder, pharmacotherapy benefits most patients. Second, although a patient with a mild depression may have psychologic factors involved in this symptomatology, it does not rule out the possible value of pharmacotherapy. The physician must expect a large number of treatment failures in such cases, but it pays to try drug therapy in this group because some patients will respond. Physicians become discouraged with pharmacotherapy when they have not made the distinction between severely depressed patients, most of whom will respond to treatment, and mildly depressed patients, most of whom will not respond. I hope that with research on some of the newer diagnostic systems, we will be able to identify more clearly the 25% of mildly depressed patients who will respond to drug treatment.

Dunner: We conducted studies on stress-induced depressions. Most clinicians assume that if a patient has multiple stresses, it is the reason for the affective disorder. However, in our studies there was very poor correlation between stress and depression. To us, this means a patient who has many stresses will not necessarily benefit more from psychologic treatment than from antidepressant medication.

Katz: We must remember not to deal in extremes. At one time, we explained all depression on the basis of psychoanalytic theory. This was wrong. We didn't know then about neurotransmitters and other chemicals presumably involved in the process. Now we must not go to the other extreme, explaining all depressions on the basis of some genetic or internal biochemical aberration. Certainly, there are many societary reasons for depression and we should balance the two. We must realize that while biochemistry can play an important role in the etiology of depression, psychologic factors are always involved. Therefore, let's take the concept of "psychobiology" seriously.

Unipolar and Bipolar Depression: Recent Findings from Clinical and Biologic Studies

David L. Dunner

Harborview Medical Center; Department of Psychiatry and Behavioral Sciences, University of Washington, Seattle, Washington

The separation of affective states into unipolar and bipolar subtypes was proposed by *Leonhard* et al. [1], and subsequent support for the separation was provided by data from depression research centers in both Europe and the United States. These studies were reviewed in 1975 by *Fieve and Dunner* [2]. The evidence supporting the unipolar-bipolar classification of affective disorder was separated into clinical, biologic, pharmacologic, and genetic studies. Bipolar patients (compared with unipolars) tended to have an early age of onset (mean 28 years), cyclic depressions, higher frequency of postpartum onsets, retarded depressions, and a greater tendency for suicide attempts. Unipolar patients' mean age of onset was 36 years; they tended to have single episodes, their depressions being often confounded with anxiety [3–6] (tables I, II).

Table I. Bipolar-unipolar distinctions (data prior to 1976)

Clinical	BP	UP
Age (years)	early (28)	late (36)
Course	cyclic	single episode
Postpartum onset	high	low
Mental status	psychomotor retardation	agitation/anxiety
Suicide attempts	high	low

Biologic studies (tables III, IV) revealed that bipolar and unipolar patients showed significant differences in EEG-measured cortical-evoked response, urinary 17-hydroxycorticosteroid excretion, mean activity of erythrocyte catechol-*o*-methyltransferase (COMT), and mean activity of platelet monoamine oxidase (MAO). Studies of central nervous system dopamine, using the proben-

Table II. Unipolar-bipolar classification (current data)

Clinical	BPI	BPII	UP
Age of onset	31	35	41
% rapid cyclers	13	16	0
Psychomotor retardation	1.9	1.0	1.0
Depression ratings, patients	30.0	22.6	31.2
Depression ratings, nurses	22.9	25.9	29.2
Reactivity	+	++	0
Borderline	+	++	0
MPI–extraversion	27.0	27.6	21.3
Suicide history, %	33.3	45.3	35.4

Table III. Bipolar-unipolar distinctions (data prior to 1976)

Biologic	BP	UP
AER	augmentor	reducer
17-OHCS (urine)	low	normal
COMT activity	low (women)	lower (women)
MAO activity	low	normal
Dopamine turnover	high	low

Table IV. Unipolar-bipolar classification (current data)

Biologic	BPI	BPII	UP
AER	augmentor	augmentor	reducer
COMT (females)	4.82	5.51	4.56
MAO	5.54	6.59	4.94
TSH to TRH	12.3		4.0
MHPG (approximate)	1,000		1,400
Li RBC/pl.	0.51	0.50	0.38
Li pump	0.24	0.25	0.25

ecid technique, revealed higher turnover of dopamine in bipolar than in unipolar patients [7–11].

Pharmacologic studies (tables V, VI) indicated that an antidepressant response to lithium during acute depression was seen more frequently among bipolar than unipolar patients [12, 13]. *L*-Dihydroxyphenylalanine levodopa ad-

Table V. Bipolar-unipolar distinctions (data prior to 1976)

Pharmacologic	BP	UP
Lithium	antimanic	no acute effect
L-Dopa	psychosis	no effect
L-Tryptophan	antidepressant	no effect

Table VI. Unipolar-bipolar classification (current data)

Pharmacologic	BPI	BPII	UP
Lithium–antidepressant	+	+	0
L-Tryptophan–antidepressant	+	+	0

Table VII. Bipolar-unipolar distinctions (data prior to 1976)

Genetic	BP	UP
Psychosis	high	lower
Suicide	high	lower
Mania	present	absent
Depression	present	present
MR aff. dis.	high (40%)	low (10–15%)
Transmission	X-linked	?

Table VIII. Unipolar-bipolar classification (current data)

Genetic	BPI	BPII	UP
Assortative mating	+	+	0
FH B1,[1]%	8	2	0
FH B2,[1]%	15	15	5
FH UP,[1]%	20	20	10

[1] Approximate morbid risks.

ministration produced psychosis or a manic-like response in bipolar patients compared with unipolar depressive patients [14, 15]. *L*-Tryptophan may also result in differential responses [16].

Data from genetic studies (tables VII, VIII) provided the earliest support for the unipolar-bipolar distinction, and these data have for the most part been confirmed in subsequent studies. *Leonhard* et al. [1] reported a higher incidence of psychosis and suicide among relatives of bipolar compared with unipolar patients. *Perris* [17] found bipolar illness among relatives of bipolar probands and little unipolar illness. He defined unipolar as three separate depressive episodes. In this study, *Perris* [17] reports that relatives of unipolar probands had unipolar illness and little bipolar illness. Similar results for unipolars were reported by *Angst* [18], who found that relatives of bipolar probands had high morbidity risks for both unipolar and bipolar illness. The difference between the *Perris* [17] and *Angst* [18] findings seems mainly the result of their respective definitions of unipolar illness.

Winokur et al. [3] reported family study data showing high morbid risks for bipolar and unipolar illness among relatives of bipolar patients, and they proposed that bipolar illness might be transmitted by a gene on the X chromosome. Their genetic studies of unipolar patients suggested that there could be at least two types of unipolar illness—"depression spectrum disease" (women with an early age of onset who had family histories of depression and alcoholism) and "pure depressive disease" (men with a late age of onset whose relatives had depression but no increase in the morbid risk of alcoholism) [19].

Thus, by 1975 a considerable amount of data had accumulated to support the biopolar-unipolar classification. Work by *Dunner* et al. [6] proposed a subclassification of bipolar and unipolar illness. They noted that the severity of mania could be used to separate patients into two groups: bipolar I (patients who had severe mania documented by hospitalization for mania) and bipolar II (patients whose severity of mania did not result in such significant social disruption or hospitalization). Bipolar II patients were often classified as unipolar by investigators because their clinical course was characterized by recurrent depression and their hypomanic episodes often seemed to be of social and clinical benefit. However, as discussed in the review by *Fieve and Dunner* [2], when data of bipolar II patients were analyzed separately from data of bipolar I and unipolar patients, it appeared that bipolar II patients shared clinical characteristics with unipolar patients but showed pharmacologic and genetic similarities to bipolar I patients.

The purpose of this paper is to discuss the current status of the bipolar-unipolar classification of affective disorders, with particular reference to research conducted in the 5 years since the review by *Fieve and Dunner* [2]. The accrued clinical, biologic, and pharmacologic data will be emphasized. The genetic studies to support the classification have not, as of this date, been reported except for preliminary analyses. Areas for future research and research strategies will be discussed.

Clinical Studies

The age of onset differences reported in the early studies have been confirmed [20]. Considering the age at first treatment as the age of onset, bipolar illness is symptomatic earlier in life than unipolar illness. Patients classified as bipolar II have an intermediate age of onset compared with other subjects. As an index of episode frequency, the incidence of rapid cycling (4 or more episodes per year) was examined among patients attending a lithium clinic. About 10–15% of bipolar I and II patients had evidence of rapid cycling, whereas none of the unipolar patients had high episode frequencies [21]. Psychomotor retardation as an important indicator of bipolar I depression has been confirmed [22]. Furthermore, it appears that bipolar II depressed patients may differ from other depressives as to their ability to mask their depression. In examining depression ratings, bipolar II patients were likely to rate themselves as more depressed compared with the nurses' ratings of their depression. This is in contrast to other primary depressives, whose self-ratings revealed less severe depression than nurses' ratings. Thus, raters are likely to misjudge the severity of depression as experienced by bipolar II patients. It is possible that this phenomenon may contribute to the increased suicide behavior in bipolar II patients. Furthermore, depressed bipolar II patients often become clinically elated when discussing their past hypomanic episodes. This affective reactivity may be related to the clinical masking of depression often seen among bipolar II patients, and also may contribute to their suicidal behavior.

Although borderline personality features have not been systematically studied in primary affective disorder, the data from *Akiskal* et al. [23] suggest that there should be a significant overlap of borderline personality and bipolar II. *Akiskal* et al. [23] found that patients with cyclothymic disorder have a high incidence of promiscuous behavior, marital failure, financial disaster, unstable employment records, and drug and alcohol abuse. Cyclothymic, as defined by *Akiskal* et al. [23], is practically identical with bipolar II as defined by *Dunner* et al.[6].

Other personality traits have been studied in bipolar and unipolar depressive patients. *Liebowitz* et al. [24] administered the Maudsley Personality Inventory and the Marke Nyman Temperament Scale to a group of outpatient depressives. Significant differences were noted on the extraversion scale. Bipolars showed more extraversion than unipolars, as expected. Lower neuroticism scores were seen in bipolar I and bipolar II patients compared with unipolar patients. However, when only those patients strictly defined as euthymic were considered, these personality measurement differences were not significant.

That is, some of the scales used to measure personality actually reflected mood states of patients and should be considered state rather than trait measures. Regarding the Marke Nyman Temperament Scale, no significant differences were found among affectively ill subtypes.

The higher suicide attempt frequency in bipolar compared with unipolar patients has been confirmed. Furthermore, bipolar II patients had higher suicide attempt frequencies than other affectively ill subtypes [25].

Biologic Studies

It was hoped that the continued demonstration of biologic and pharmacologic differences between unipolar and bipolar patients would ultimately lead toward a hypothesis regarding the presumed biologic basis of these disorders. It appeared that neuroendocrine and enzymatic dysfunction, as reported in the earlier studies, might suggest an amine transmitter basis for the disorder. Supporting data were derived from the differential effects of levodopa in depressed subtypes. Biopolar I depressives developed psychosis, bipolar II depressives demonstrated an antidepressant response, and unipolar patients showed no effect [15].

Few attempts at replicating prior studies have been reported, however, and some results have not been reproduced. For example, the work of *Buchsbaum* et al. [7], noting that bipolar patients (types 1 and 2) were augmentors and unipolars were reducers (as shown by average cortical-evoked response), has been replicated [26]. However, the reported differences in mean activities of enzymes (COMT and MAO) have not been consistently replicated in the studies of several groups [27–30]. Further, attempts to replicate the probenecid data regarding central nervous system turnover of dopamine have not been reported.

Gold et al. [31] reported bipolar-unipolar differences in the thyroid stimulating hormone (TSH) response to thyrotropin-releasing hormone (TRH), with unipolar depressed patients having a significantly lower response than bipolar-depressed subjects. They also noted that 24-hour urinary free cortisol production was significantly elevated among unipolar depressives compared with controls, and *Gold* et al. [31] suggested that some unipolar depressives might have increased functional serotonergic activity. However, the dexamethasone suppression test, which was initially reported as showing unipolar-bipolar distinction [32], was more recently reported *not* to show unipolar-bipolar differences [33]. Furthermore, this test, which can differentiate primary depressives with endogenomorphic features from other depressives, can be demonstrated only while patients are symptomatic. It is likely that a true biologic test, able to differentiate bipolar from unipolar depression, will not be state dependent.

Studies of the urinary excretion of 3-methoxy-4-hydroxphenylglycol (MHPG), a norepinephrine metabolite, seem to show consistent differences with bipolar depressives having lower mean excretion than unipolar depressives [34]. However, the relationship of *urinary* MHPG to *central nervous system* neurotransmitter function has not been clearly elucidated. It is quite possible that the differences in mean urinary MHPG excretion reflect physical activity (bipolars having greater psychomotor retardation than unipolars) rather than central functions.

Pharmacologic studies have largely confirmed the antidepressant effect of lithium carbonate among bipolar compared with unipolar patients [35]. Preliminary reports on a few patients suggest that bipolar depressives may be more likely to have an antidepressant response to *L*-tryptophan than unipolar patients [36]. To our knowledge, there has been no attempt to replicate the differential effects of levodopa in bipolar and unipolar depressive patients [15]. Furthermore, no controlled data exist regarding comparative effects of tricyclic antidepressants and MAO inhibitors in bipolar versus unipolar depressives.

Interest in lithium metabolism in erythrocytes has resulted in a series of research reports [37–41]. Earlier suggestions that unipolar-bipolar differences in lithium red blood cell : plasma ratio were related to diagnosis were not supported by subsequent studies, which related the lithium erythocyte : plasma ratio to plasma lithium concentrations [37–40]. Furthermore, studies of lithium erythrocyte transport have also failed to show differences in unipolar compared with bipolar patients [41].

Genetic Studies

Clearly, there are important and consistent genetic differences between bipolar and unipolar patients. At least two extensive family investigations of the genetics of depression were undertaken in the 1970s, and the completed analysis of these data is awaited with interest. Preliminary data from the New York Study (New York State Psychiatric Institute, Columbia University, The Foundation of Depression and Manic Depression) reveal that bipolar I illness is found in families of bipolar I and bipolar II patients, but not in families of unipolar patients [42]. These data support the notion that bipolar I illness is inherited and that bipolar II patients are genetically bipolar and not unipolar. Furthermore, the New York data indicate that the morbid risk for primary affective disorder among first-degree relatives of bipolar I probands is about 40%, most of this illness being unipolar rather than bipolar. Thus, some unipolar individuals presumably have a bipolar genotype, (i.e., are from families with mania). Genetic analyses of the mode of transmission are in progress. Preliminary data do not suggest that either X chromosome linkage or a single Mendelian dominant form of transmission is involved [42].

The heritability of bipolar illness has led to a new area of research: biogenetics. This research tests biologic and pharmacologic factors in relatives of patients with depression, in the hope of determining the suitability of these factors as genetic markers. This area was recently reviewed by *Gershon* [43], who noted that the validity of a genetic marker has two requirements: the identification of a homogeneous population on the basis of clinical, biologic, and pharmacologic characteristics, and the relation of the marker to transmission of the disorder within families.

In searching for state-independent markers of bipolar illness, enzymes involved in amine metabolism and lithium transport systems have been extensively studied [29, 30, 41]. However, these potential markers (MAO, COMT, the "lithium pump") have not proved fruitful as markers for the disorder, even though MAO and the lithium pump may be under genetic control [29, 47]. In reviewing the data regarding erythrocyte COMT, we noted that differences were found in the mean activity of COMT for bipolar compared with unipolar patients. However, these differences were not confirmed by studies at multiple centers [30]. It was suggested that demonstrating differences in mean activity of enzymes, where the range of values overlaps between bipolars and unipolars, may produce statistically significant but not biologically meaningful data presumably because of sampling errors. Hemoglobin electrophoresis, as a test for hemoglobin S in patients with sickle cell anemia and their families, is a medical prototype of the biogenetic studies being undertaken in psychiatry. Unfortunately, we are not finding abnormal enzyme activity in the groups under study. However, one center may report a positive finding (for example with MAO) which is not replicated by a second center. This type of nonreplication suggests that we have not yet studied the appropriate marker. It is possible that the genetic analysis of the New York data may point toward linkage with an autosomal marker and suggest a mode of transmission for the illness. These data are awaited within interest.

Summary of Research

The differentiation of bipolar from unipolar depressive patients has received continual support from clinical studies. The separation of bipolar II patients from other primary affective disorder subtypes has not been supported by research data to the extent that bipolar II has become an acceptable subgroup. Nonetheless, the additional research studies have pointed toward the establishment of bipolar II as a meaningful subtype. The pharmacologic and biologic studies in the past 5 years have not, in the main, extended the data supporting the bipolar-unipolar distinction. Genetic data, which were the basis for the initial separation of depressed patients into unipolar and bipolar types, are in the process of being analyzed. The genetic data may provide a useful basis for understanding where bipolar II patients fit into the unipolar-bipolar schema.

At the present time no single test, sign, or symptom, or group of tests, signs, or symptoms exists which permits clear differentiation of unipolar depressives from bipolar depressives. It is hoped that continued research will lead toward a true measurement of the correct variable and that this will point toward the etiology of these disorders.

From a clinical point of view it is believed that affective illness, and bipolar illness in particular, accounts for many of the patients previously diagnosed as schizophrenic but showing either episodic courses or affective (particularly manic) symptoms. Thus, many patients with atypical symptoms and atypical courses of illness are given the clinical label of bipolar illness, perhaps in the hope that the label will make such patients responsive to lithium treatment. Suffice it to say the the research studies supporting the bipolar-unipolar distinction were based on patients defined in such a rigorous way that fairly homogeneous groups emerged. Clinicians should be cautious in relabeling patients in the absence of criteria necessary for the diagnosis of bipolar or unipolar depression, or in the presence of exclusion criteria (such as polydrug abuse).

Although much work has been done using the unipolar-bipolar classification, the dichotomy is not uniformly accepted by researchers. The proposed new nomenclature (DSMIII) makes reference to the unipolar-bipolar classification. However, affective disorders in DSMIII are classified according to a system which seems to lack the validation provided as a basis either for the criteria of *Feighner* et al. [44] or for the unipolar-bipolar classification. Thus, future depression research on unipolars may include some patients who would have been excluded by the *Feighner* et al. [44] criteria as secondary depressions, but who meet the DSMIII criteria of major affective disorders. Furthermore, bipolar I defines manic depressives more strictly than the DSMIII major affective disorder with mania. Thus, use of DSMIII may result in less homogeneity in affectively ill populations. The impact of this relative diagnostic imprecision on the psychiatric literature is problematic.

Areas for Future Research

Patients with a history of hallucinogenic drug abuse sometimes appear to have a bipolar disorder. The clinical description of this secondary bipolar illness, and determination of appropriate treatment, is a fruitful area of research. Further work is also needed to differentiate unipolar subtypes as in the model proposed by *Baker* et al. [19].

There are several pharmacologic studies of interest. A well-controlled study of the comparative efficacy of tricyclic antidepressants in unipolar compared with bipolar patients is clearly indicated for both acute depression and prophylaxis for depression. Studies of other pharmacologic agents, such as *L*-tryptophan in acute depression, are also warranted. The dexamethasone suppression test provides an interesting biologic dichotomy of depressed patients. It would seem reasonable to attempt correlating results from this test with other variables, such as tricyclic antidepressant response and family history.

The major area of genetic research in depression in the 1980s will undoubtedly be in the area of "high risk" studies. These will follow from early ages children of patients with unipolar and bipolar depression. If the early manifestations of bipolar and unipolar disorders can be detected, then appropriate treatment could be instituted to prevent the full clinical expression of the disorder. Such high risk studies truly encompass clinical, biologic and genetic designs. This is because the clinical signs should correlate with appropriate biologic markers, to permit earlier identifications of individuals at risk for development of illness. These studies may be particularly fruitful in families with bipolar illness because genetic factors seem to be important in the etiology of bipolar mood disorders.

Research in depression is broadly based, and there is considerable research interest in life stress, cross-cultural phenomena, and effects of aging, as well as in the biologic and genetic components of unipolar and bipolar depressions. It is hoped that these future studies will provide a rational basis for classification and therapy of these disorders.

References

1   Leonhard, K.; Korff, I.; Shulz, H.: Die Temperamente in den Familien der monopolaren und bipolaren phasichen Psychosen. Psychiat. Neurol. *143:* 416–434 (1962).

2   Fieve, R.R.; Dunner, D.L.: Unipolar and bipolar affective states; in Flack, Draghi, The nature and treatment of depression (Wiley, New York 1975).
3   Winokur, G.; Clayton, P.; Reich, T.: Manic depressive illness (Mosby, St. Louis 1969).
4   Dunner, D.L.; Fieve, R.R.: Clinical factors in lithium carbonate prophylaxis failure. Archs. gen. Psychiat. *30:* 229–233 (1974).
5   Beigel, A.; Murphy, D.L.: Unipolar and bipolar affective illness: differences in clinical characteristics accompanying depression. Archs. gen. Psychiat. *24:* 215–229 (1971).
6   Dunner, D.L.; Gershon, E.S.; Goodwin, F.K.: Heritable factors in the severity of affective illness. Sci. Proc. Am. psychiat. Ass. *123:* 187–188 (1970).
7   Buchsbaum, M.; Goodwin, F.K.; Murphy, D.L.; et al.: Average evoked response in affective disorders. Am. J. Psychiat. *128:* 19–25 (1971).
8   Dunner, D.L.; Gerson, E.S.; Goodwin, F.K.; et al.: Excretion of 17-hydroxycorticosteroids in unipolar and bipolar depressed patients. Archs. gen. Psychiat. *26:* 364–366 (1972).
9   Dunner, D.L.; Cohn, C.K.; Gershon, E.S.; et al.: Differential catechol-O-methyltransferase activity in unipolar and bipolar affective illness. Archs. gen. Psychiat. *25:* 348–353 (1971).
10 Murphy, D.L.; Weiss, R.: Reduced monoamine oxidase activity in blood platelets from bipolar depressed patients. Am. J. Psychiat. *128:* 1351–1357 (1972).
11 Goodwin, F.; Post, R.M.; Dunner, D.L.; et al.: Cerebrospinal fluid amine metabolites in affective illness: the probenecid technique. Am. J. Psychiat. *130:* 73–79 (1973).
12 Goodwin, F.K.; Murphy, D.L.; Dunner, D.L.; et al.: Lithium response in unipolar versus bipolar depression. Am. J. Psychiat. *129:* 44–47 (1972).
13 Mendels, J.; Secunda, S.K.; Dyson, W.L.: A controlled study of the antidepressant effects of lithium carbonate. Archs. gen. Psychiat. *26:* 154–157 (1972).
14 Murphy, D.L.; Brodie, H.K.H.; Goodwin, F.K.; et al.: Regular induction of hypomania by *L*-dopa in bipolar manic-depressive patients. Nature, Lond. *229:* 135–136 (1971).
15 Gershon, E.S.; Bunney, W.E., Jr.; Goodwin, F.K.; et al.: Catecholamines and affective illness: studies with *L*-dopa and alpha-methyl-para-tyrosine; in Ho, McIsaac, Brain chemistry and mental disease, pp. 135–161 (Plenum Press, New York 1971).
16 Murphy, D.L.; Baker, M.; Goodwin, F.K.; et al.: *L*-Tryptophan in affective disorders: indoleamine changes and differential clinical effects. Psychopharmacologia *34:* 11–20 (1964).
17 Perris, C.: A study of bipolar (manic-depressive) and unipolar recurrent depressive psychoses. Acta psychiat. scand. *42:* suppl. 194 (1966).
18 Angst, J.: Zur Ätiologie und Nosologie endogener depressive Psychosen; in Monographien aus dem Gesamtgebiete der Neurologie und Psychiatrie (Springer, Berlin 1966).
19 Baker, M.; Dorzab, J.; Winokur, G.; et al.: Depressive disease: classification and clinical characteristics. Compreh. Psychiat. *12:* 354–365 (1971).

20 Dunner, D.L.; Gershon, E.S.; Goodwin, F.K.: Heritable factors in the severity of affective illness. Biol. Psychiat. 11: 31–42 (1976).
21 Dunner, D.L.; Patrick, V.; Fieve, R.R.: Rapid cycling manic depressive patients. Compreh. Psychiat. *18:* 561–566 (1977).
22 Dunner, D.L.; Dwyer, T.; Fieve, R.R.: Depressive symptoms in patients with unipolar and bipolar affective disorder. Compreh. Psychiat. *17:* 447–451 (1976).
23 Akiskal, H.S.; Djenderedjian, A.H.; Rosenthal, R.H.; et al.: Cyclothymic disorder: validating criteria for inclusion in the bipolar affective group. Am. J. Psychiat. *135:* 1227–1233 (1977).
24 Liebowitz, M.R.; Stallone, F.; Dunner, D.L.; Fieve, R.R.: Personality features of patients with primary affective disorder. Acta psychiat. scand. *60:* 214–224 (1979).
25 Stallone, F.; et al.: Personal communication (1980).
26 Buchsbaum, M.S.; Lavine, R.A.; Davis, G.C.; et al.: Effects of lithium on somatosensory-evoked potentials and prediction of clinical response in patients with affective illness. International Lithium Conference: Controversies and unresolved issues, New York 1978. (in press, 1980).
27 Gershon, E.S.; Jonas, W.Z.: Erythrocyte-soluble catechol-O-methyltransferase activity in primary affective disorder. Archs. gen. Psychiat. *32:* 1351–1356 (1975).
28 Mattsson, B.; Mjorndal, T.; Oreland, L.; et al.: Catechol-O-methyltransferase and plasma monoamine oxidase in patients with affective disorders. Acta psychiat. scand. *225:* suppl., p. 187 (1974).
29 Fieve, R.R.; Kumbaraci, T.; Kassir, S.; et al.: Platelet monoamine oxidase activity in affective disorder. Biol. Psychiat. (in press, 1980).
30 Dunner, D.L.; Levitt, M.; Kumbaraci, T.; et al.: Erythrocyte catechol-O-methyltransferase activity in primary affective disorder. Biol. Psychiat. *12:* 237–244 (1977).
31 Gold, P.W.; Goodwin, F.K.; Wehr, T.; et al.: Pituitary thyrotropin response to thyrotropin-releasing hormone in affective illness: relationship to spinal fluid amine metabolites. Am. J. Psychiat. *134:* 1028–1031 (1977).
32 Carroll, B.J.; Curtis, G.C.; Mendels, J.: Neuroendocrine regulation in depression. I. Discrimination of depressed from nondepressed patients. Archs. gen. Psychiat. *33:* 1051–1058 (1976).
33 Carroll, B.: Neuroendocrine diagnostic criteria for depression. Annual Meeting American College of Neuropsychopharmacology, San Juan, Puerto Rico (1979).
34 Schildkraut, J.J.: Current status of the catecholamine hypothesis of affective disorders; in Lipton, Mascio, Killam, Psychopharmacology: a generation of progress (Raven Press, New York 1978).
35 Dunner, D.L.; Fieve, R.R.: The effect of lithium in depressive subtypes; in Deniker, Radouco-Thomas, Villeneuve, Neuropsychopharmacology, pp. 1109–1115 (Pergamon Press, New York 1978).
36 Farkas, T.; Dunner, D.L.; Fieve, R.R.: *L*-Tryptophan in depression. Biol. Psychiat. *11:* 295–302 (1976).
37 Mendels, J.; Frazer, A.: Intracellular lithium concentration and clinical response: towards a membrane theory of depression. J. psychiat. Res. *10:* 9–18 (1973).

38   Lyttkens, L.; Soderberg, U.; Wetterberg, L.: Increased lithium erythrocyte/plasma ratio in manic-depressive psychosis. Lancet *i:* 40 (1973).
39   Kim, Y.B.; Dunner, D.L.; Meltzer, H.L.; et al.: Lithium erythrocyte: plasma ratio in primary affective disorder. Am. Psychiat. *19:* 129–134 (1978).
40   Schreiner, H.C.; Dunner, D.L.; Meltzer, H.L.; et al.: The relationship of the lithium erythrocyte : plasma ratio to plasma lithium level. Biol. Psychiat. *14:* 207–213 (1979).
41   Dunner, D.L.; Meltzer, H.L.; Fieve, R.R.: Clinical correlates of the lithium pump. Am. J. Psychiat. *135:* 1062–1064 (1978).
42   Go, R.; Dunner, D.L.; Fieve, R.R.: Comparison of autosomal dominant and X-linked dominant models to a set of sixty-five bipolar proband families. Annual Meeting Psychiatric Research Society, Madison, WI 1979.
43   Gershon, E.S.: The search for genetic markers in affective disorders; in Lipton, DiMascio, Killam, Psychopharmacology: a generation of progress (Raven Press, New York 1978).
44   Feighner, J.P.; Robins, E.; Guze, S.B.; et al.: Diagnostic criteria for use in psychiatric research. Archs. gen. Psychiat. *26:* 57–63 (1972).

Discussion

Maas: In addition to classifying patients as bipolar II if they have a history of hypomania, some investigators say patients are bipolar II if they have a drug-induced hypomania. Do you agree?

Dunner: Yes. Tricyclic-induced hypomania counts. However, our data show that this is unusual in patients who don't have a history of mania. Interestingly, *Abrams and Taylor* found that patients with tricyclic-induced hypomania also seem to have a history of hypomania.

Maas: Given the diagnosis of bipolar type II, the issue becomes one of prophylaxis. The data suggest that bipolar patients should receive lithium therapy, but I worry about its renal toxicity and its appropriateness in bipolar II patients.

Dunner: It's clear that bipolar I patients who, for example, experience two episodes of mania in an 8-year period should receive prophylactic lithium therapy. Bipolar II patients often are called unipolars because they present with complaints of recurrent depression and not of hypomania. From some preliminary studies, using small groups of bipolar II patients, it appeared that lithium and placebo show no difference in effect after 16 months' administration. Looking at the data from these patients after 2½ years' treatment, we noticed a decrease in the frequency of depressive episodes in the lithium group. The dropout rate was significantly different between the two groups. More patients taking placebo dropped out of the study. I think lithium had an antidepressive effect and elicited a prophylactic response in these bipolar II patients.

Maas: If bipolar II patients are given a tricyclic drug rather than lithium, do they have the same incidence of hypomanic episodes as the manic patient?

Dunner: I believe they do.

Janowsky: Are you convinced that lithium is of no value in unipolar depression?

Dunner: Yes.

Janowsky: What do you mean by family history? Where do you draw the line?

Dunner: Family history data refer to first-degree relatives, i.e., parents and siblings. It does not include grandparents, aunts, uncles, etc. For our family studies, we interviewed first-degree relatives in addition to the patient. About 70% of our patients had a family history of depression in their first-degree relatives. Theoretically, if we included second-degree relatives in our study, the morbidity risk would drop by half.

Mendels: Research data suggest that lithium is an effective antidepressant in some patients, but lithium is not approved as an antidepressant by the Food and Drug Administration. We don't want to leave the impression that it should be used as such on a widespread basis. From a practical standpoint, we know that in treating bipolar patients, lithium, although an antidepressant, is not a perfect antidepressant for all such patients. In general, we treat a bipolar depressed patient with a tricyclic drug while administering lithium at the same time to reduce the risk of a tricyclic-precipitated manic or hypomanic episode.

Dunner: A number of physicians overdiagnose manic depressive illness and use lithium inappropriately. For example, individuals with extensive polydrug histories who have somewhat transient bipolar mood swings are being called manic-depressives and are given lithium. Sometimes, clinicians confuse amphetamine psychosis and PCP psychosis with mania and prescribe lithium. We must be alert to this.

The Psychobiology of Affective Disorders. Pfizer Symp. Depression, Boca Raton 1980, pp. 25–39 (Karger, Basel 1980)

Genetic Factors from a Clinical Perspective

Elliot S. Gershon

Section on Psychogenetics, Biological Psychiatry Branch, National Institute of Mental Health, Bethesda, Maryland

Introduction

The idea of genetic differences in the emotional vulnerabilities and intellectual capacities of people has been accepted with reluctance among mental health professionals. One reason for resisting the idea in psychiatric illnesses is the fear that it will induce therapeutic nihilism and promote stigmatization of the victims of illness. In this paper, I will refer briefly to the evidence that genetic factors are of crucial importance in determining vulnerability to major affective disorder. The emphasis of the paper will be on the valuable and useful implications of current genetic knowledge for the characterization, treatment, and secondary prevention of these disorders. Let me caution at the outset that although our knowledge has advanced, it is still limited. We still do not have a test for genetic vulnerability that we can give to any individual, nor a precise characterization of the mode of inheritance of the affective disorders.

Evidence for Genetic Factors

Identical and fraternal twins have common environments, but fraternal twins share only part of their genetic makeup whereas identical twins share all of it. Thus, the consistent finding that approximately 65% of identical twins will be concordant for major affective disorder, versus 14% concordance in fraternal twins, implies that genetic vulnerability is playing a major role [1]. Further evidence favoring genetic transmission of vulnerability to major affective illness is found in the adoption study of bipolar illness performed by *Mendelwicz and Rainer* [2], and *Kety* [3], who studied suicide in biologic relatives of depressed adoptees.

Other points can be illustrated by twin data. The finding that about 20% of concordant identical twins have different forms of mood disorder, where one is unipolar and the other is bipolar, indicates that in some cases these two disorders are manifestations of the same genetic vulnerability. The considerable proportion of identical twins who are not concordant suggests that either some cases of illness are phenocopies (illness found in the absence of genetic vulnerability to it) or there is variable penetrance. Penetrance refers to the frequency (usually a percentage) with which a mutant gene produces its effect in those persons possessing it. A gene with low penetrance refers to a gene which will show its effect or produce illness in 10–20% of those who have the gene. A third point is that the twin studies, which strongly support heritability of both unipolar and bipolar illness, were all done with severely ill patients, so that we may not be able to generalize this evidence for milder forms of depression.

Clinical Subdivisions of Affective Disorders

The bipolar-unipolar distinction in affective disorders, originally proposed by *Leonhard* [4] and *Leonhard* et al. [5], is the most widely known clinical subdivision of the affective disorders. Bipolar patients are those who have had both manic and depressive episodes, while unipolar patients have had only depression. Unipolar manics are included with bipolar illness by virtually all investigators [6].

The widely accepted bipolar-unipolar difference in illness distribution in relatives of patients with these two types of disorders led *Leonhard* and some later investigators to consider these disorders as genetically distinct (fig. 1). The families of bipolar patients have increased total morbidity (increased bipolar and increased unipolar illness) compared with families of unipolar patients. In earlier studies, the relative absence of bipolar disorders in families of unipolar patients seemed to support the genetic distinctiveness of these two disorders. But even those studies showed an increased incidence of unipolar relatives in families of bipolar patients. Later studies showed, as one would expect, an increased incidence of bipolar relatives (compared with the population prevalence) for unipolar patients. Mathematical analyses showed that these family patterns were generally compatible with a single, underlying disorder producing both unipolar and bipolar illness. Bipolar illness was a genetically more severe form, in the sense that more illness was transmitted in families of bipolar than in families of unipolar patients [1]. Identical twin pairs, in which one is unipolar and the other is bipolar, provide the most convincing clinical evidence that at least a substantial proportion of patients of the two disorders are biologically

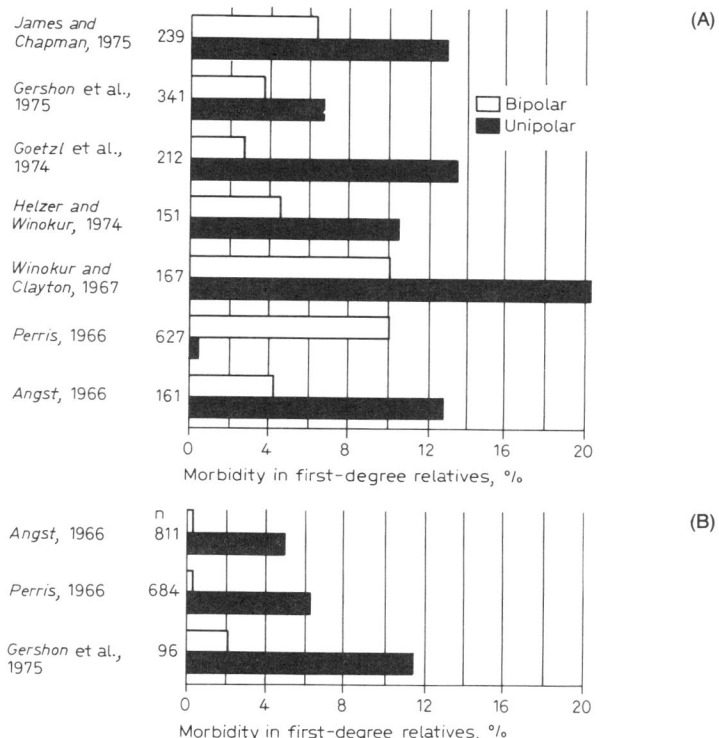

Fig. 1. Studies of first-degree relatives of both bipolar (A) and unipolar (B) patients show high incidence of affective disorders. All but one (*Perris*, fig. 1A) show higher unipolar than bipolar morbidity, and all but one (*Gershon* et al., fig. 1B) show greater risk to relatives of bipolars. These inconsistencies, as well as interstudy variations in morbidity, probably stem in part from differences in diagnostic criteria [adapted from ref. 31].
(Reprinted by permission from E.S. Gershon: "Genetics of the affective disorders," *Hospital Practice*, Vol. 14, No. 3, March 1979. New York: HP Publishing Co. Figure by A. Miller.)

and genetically equivalent, as noted above. I have reviewed the numerous biologic and pharmacologic differences reported in initial studies of bipolar and unipolar patients which were not consistently replicated later on. At present, the only consistently replicated finding is that bipolar patients have a more frequent acute antidepressant response to lithium carbonate (as opposed to prophylaxis, where lithium is equally valuable in both types of patients). This may be related to a genetic abnormality in membrane ion transport, as discussed below.

From the practical viewpoint of predicting risk in family members, or choice of medication, it is useful to think in terms of bipolar and related disorders. For example, *Kupfer* et al. [8] have demonstrated that the antidepressant response to lithium in unipolar patients correlates positively with family history of bipolar illness. However, there may be genetic variants of bipolar disorders and environmentally produced bipolar-like disorders. *Krauthammer and Klerman* [9] reviewed reports on nongenetic mania including drug-induced, posttraumatic and postinfectious cases. Women with postpartum mania have less often a positive family history for psychiatric illness than other manics [10] and may represent a mixture of both genetic and nongenetic cases produced by metabolic, hormonal or stressful events.

Dunner et al. [11] divided bipolar illness into patients who have had frank mania (bipolar I) and patients with a history of hypomania (bipolar II). Bipolar II patients may prove to be pharmacologically distinct. Levodopa seems to act as a satisfactory antidepressant only in this group [12]. It has been argued by *Akiskal* et al. [13] that patients with hypomania produced by antidepressant treatment should be considered bipolar II since they nearly always have *spontaneous* episodes of hypomania as well. Genetically, these patients are generally considered similar to bipolar I patients, although preliminary studies have shown differences in morbid risk among relatives [11].

In genetic research, unipolar disorder (major depressive disorder) has been defined in various ways, usually depending on the severity of the depression. *Perris* [14] required three episodes with hospitalization or medical treatment, whereas the recent NIMH collaborative study, using the Research Diagnostic Criteria [15], accepts one episode of 2 weeks' duration, characterized by depressive mood, at least four somatic symptoms of depression, and mild social or familial functional impairment. When depression is defined as a more severe disorder, including hospitalization or incapacitation, it is a relatively uncommon disorder [20]. Its lifetime prevalence in the population is 2½–6%, and it has a very strong familial concentration that fits genetic models for either single gene or multifactorial transmission [1]. When defined according to the broader Research Diagnostic Criteria, the population lifetime prevalence is estimated at 21% [16] and genetic transmission was *excluded* in a recent, careful analysis of family study data [17]. The familial influence appeared to be a sibling-sibling cultural effect (i.e., nongenetic causes of similarities between offspring). The psychiatrist making genetic counseling and treatment decisions would do well to bear these discrepancies in mind since they may define genetic and nongenetic forms of depression.

Within severe unipolar disorders, *Van Valkenburg* et al. [18] proposed a distinction between "pure familial depression," "sporadic (nonfamilial) depression," and "depression spectrum disorder" (patients with a family history of alcoholism). Depression spectrum disorder was associated with abnormalities in cortisol suppression by dexamethasone while patients were ill [19] and may have a distinct chromosomal localization (as discussed below). However, the cortisol suppression finding in this subgroup of depressed patients was not replicated in a later study [pers. commun.].

Several clinical entities are found in families of patients with major affective disorders. These may share the same genetic diathesis. They are suicide, acute psychosis (schizoaffective disorder), alcoholism, and possibly drug abuse. Suicide, a major cause of death in patients hospitalized for affective disorders, also is increased among family members [3, 20]. Schizoaffective disorder (also called acute psychosis, acute schizophrenia, atypical psychosis) occurs more often in families with bipolar affective disorder than in families with schizophrenia, although both associations exist [21]. Based on our preliminary impression of a current family study, it appears that drug abuse occurs more frequently in younger family members of patients with primary affective disorder, and possibly may represent a clinical precursor of bipolar or unipolar disorders in young people [unpubl. data].

In a recent family study [18], cyclothymic personality (loosely defined as noticeable but not dysfunctional mood alterations that persist for days to weeks, including both elevated and depressed moods), occurred more frequently in families of bipolar patients than in normal controls. On the other hand, the incidence of depressive personality was not increased in families of patients with major affective disorder. The incidence of minor depression increased, but a recent study [19] suggests that this entity cannot be diagnosed reliably.

Chromosomal Linkage Markers and Biologic Vulnerability Tests

We may confirm that a genetic illness is determined at a particular chromosomal location, or by a particular genetically controlled pathophysiologic process, by tracing the illness through an extended pedigree and observing whether the illness and the marker segregate together or independently. This is one of the few causal tests in psychiatry, and it has been applied repeatedly in attempts to find chromosomal linkage in affective disorders [7]. Two genes are linked if they are close together on the same chromosome, and tend to segregate or are transmitted together in families. Nonlinked genes segregate independently. By using a *marker gene* (i.e., a gene associated with a specific illness) one can predict, within a family, who will have that disease by determining whether the marker gene is present. The best known hypothesis states that bipolar and related disorders are transmitted as a single dominant gene, located close to the gene for color blindness on the X chromosome. It has also been hypothesized that bipolar illness is closely linked to the Xg blood group gene, another X chromosome marker, at a considerable distance from color blindness. The incompatibility of close linkage of affective disorder to both locations, and other criticisms of the evidence for linkage, were reviewed by *Gershon* et al. [1]. We have not been able to confirm that bipolar illness is linked to any of the X chromosome markers or to the HLA antigen system (on chromosome 6). From these studies we have concluded that these linkages are not generally present, although it is conceivable that the single pedigree reports of linkage are correct and that rare pedigrees exist in which color blindness is genetically linked to bipoar illness.

Pathophysiologic tests to identify vulnerability to affective disorder have been attempted. Reduced activity of platelet monoamine oxidase has been observed in bipolar affective disorder, but we recently reported that this is not a marker of genetic vulnerability to the disorder [24]. However, *Pandey* et al. [25] reported an association between affective illness in relatives and monoamine oxidase enzyme activity. Other enzymes of catecholamine metabolism (catechol-O-methyltransferase in erythrocytes and dopamine-β-hydroxylase in plasma) show no relation between enzyme activity and transmission in families. A report of decreased lithium transport out of erythrocytes in the ill relatives of bipolar patients, if replicated, may contribute to a predictive test for risk in families [23]. This finding would suggest a membrane abnormality as a genetic factor in bipolar illness.

We have reviewed these issues in greater detail elsewhere [7], concluding that, at this time, there is no marker of genetic vulnerability to affective disorders as a whole, or for a subgroup of patients, that can be confidently used in the clinical assessment of individual persons or relatives of patients.

Preventive Aspects

Secondary Prevention

It is important to recognize the real limits of prevention in the light of the current knowledge reviewed here. We know that there is greatly increased risk of affective and related disorders in families of patients compared with population prevalence, but we cannot identify individuals at risk before the onset of illness. Also, we know of no environmental manipulation, including genetic counseling, that would reduce this risk. Therefore, primary prevention, in the sense of decreasing the number of new cases of manifest disease, is not within our current capabilities.

I would make one exception to these generalizations, based on an unusual case that we saw at the NIMH several years ago. A 22-year-old woman, the identical twin of a bipolar patient, asked if she should take lithium. After our examination revealed no psychopathology, we decided not to prescribe lithium. However, we offered her and her husband information on signs of incipient mania or depression. Within 6 months she developed mania. This was promptly treated with inpatient hospitalization. Since that time, the patient has had a very good response to lithium prophylaxis. In retrospect, I believe we would have done well to consider the 65% risk (without age correction) to the identical twin of the bipolar patient. The risk would be closer to 100% with age correction. Thus, perhaps lithium treatment was indicated when the patient first consulted us. In other classes of relatives, I would not feel justified instituting prophylactic lithium treatment, and I know of no other primary prevention maneuver that seems promising.

Secondary prevention of an illness in a population is the early recognition and treatment of cases that arise, reducing their morbidity. Here, the family concentration of severe primary affective disorder offers an important opportunity for prevention. In a systematic study of first-degree relatives (parents, siblings, and offspring) and second-degree relatives (grandparents, aunts and uncles, and half-siblings) of patients with bipolar disorder, we made extensive efforts to locate and examine all relatives. This included relatives at a considerable geographic distance from the patient, and those who had little knowledge of or interaction with the patient. In first-degree relatives, we found the expected high incidence of affective disorders (comparable to our previous studies), which was considerably higher than the population prevalence (table I).

Genetic Counseling

Generally, the onset of affective illness is in young adulthood. This creates different needs for genetic counseling than disorders manifest as birth defects [29]. The incipient or possible future illness in a teenage or young adult relative of a patient is the most frequent concern of persons seeking genetic counseling. The next most frequent concern, in relation to affective disorders, is whether to have children. The empirical risk for the disorder usually is not considered prohibitively high by patients and their spouses (either before or after counseling), and these individuals usually reproduce. Except in the case of

Table 1. Illness in first-degree relatives of 86 bipolar I patients [30]

	Ill, %	Alive and ill, %	Alive and ill untreated, %	No information about treatment, %
Affective disorders				
Bipolar I and bipolar II	5.9	6.1	1.2	0.2
Unipolar	10.4	11.1	2.7	1.0
Minor depression	5.0	5.7	2.0	1.2
Cyclothymic	2.1	2.8	1.0	0.5
Depressive personality	1.8	1.7	1.0	0.5
Behavioral disorders				
Sociopathy, drug abuse, alcoholism, sexual deviation	5.2	4.9	2.0	1.7
Minor emotional disorders				
Obsessive compulsive disorder, generalized anxiety disorder, panic disorder, Briquet's disorder, other psychiatric disorder without hospitalization	1.5	2.0	0.5	2.0
Major disorders				
Schizophrenia, schizoaffective disorder, unspecified functional psychosis; other psychiatric disorder with hospitalization	2.3	1.5	0.2	0.7

Note: There are 405 living and 105 dead first-degree relatives. Percentage ill not corrected for age.

clinically unmanageable affective disorder, which makes the parental role impossible to assume, I do not advise patients against having children. Since only 15% of our bipolar patients at NIMH have a bipolar parent, even from a hardheaded primary prevention viewpoint this is not necessary.

For the psychiatrist, genetic counseling is best considered as subsumed under psychotherapy. The first goal is a realistic and appropriate appreciation of the patient's own family history and of the risk to relatives. Second, one must provide a means with which to cope with the anxiety and narcissistic injury of the knowledge of genetic risk. Third, one must make appropriate plans to respond to the risk, which means early treatment for relatives beginning to show signs of mood disorder.

How can one estimate the risk to the person seeking counseling? Generally, we use the empirical risk estimates (fig. 1), assuming that they are halved for each degree of removal of the known ill relative from the person seeking counseling. But it is most important to take a very careful family history, preferably with sources of information other than just the person seeking counseling. Extensive multigeneration pedigrees are uncovered in a distinct minority of patients (fig. 2). In those cases, I believe the risk should be considered greater than the general risk to siblings or offspring, although it is a matter of inspecting and interpreting each pedigree to give an estimate of the risk. Although I have never observed such a pedigree, and am not convinced that it exists, the presence of known color blindness in a pedigree, strongly suggesting X chromosome transmission, might be used to predict risks more precisely. However, here one would have to perform a complete pedigree study, including examination of relatives for illness and color blindness, before one could be satisfied that this was a pedigree with that mode of transmission.

A second clinical use of a known family history of a major affective disorder takes a pharmacologically aggressive approach to a newly discovered illness, particularly a mild form of illness. For example, I often treat moderate depression in a late adolescent child of a patient with bipolar illness as if it

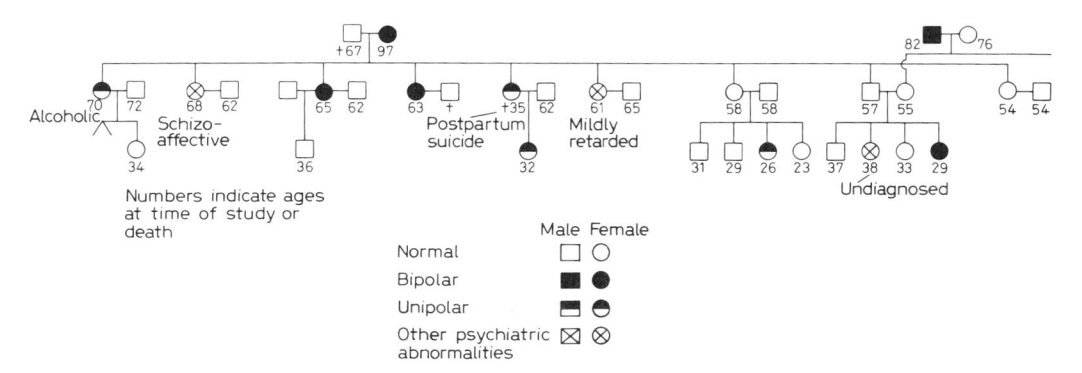

Fig. 2. This pedigree of a large family in New England exemplifies several aspects of the affective disorders in addition to their tendency to run in families. Presence of both unipolar and bipolar disorders and a case of schizoaffective disorder suggests that these conditions are etiologically related. Major affective illness is present in each of three generations of this pedigree with both consanguinity and assortative mating. The two ancestral persons are distantly related (not illustrated for space reasons). Two well persons, each having a parent with bipolar manic depressive illness, have married (a form of assortative mating) and have two daughters who have had psychiatric hospitalization, one of them with bipolar illness [adapted from ref. 31].
(Reprinted by permission from E.S. Gershon: "Genetics of the affective disorders," *Hospital Practice,* Vol. 14, No. 3, March 1979. New York: HP Publishing Co. Figure by A. Miller.)

were a major affective disorder rather than treating it as the ubiquitous developmental depressive crisis of late adolescence.

Finally, in counseling situations we must consider the patient's spouse. A tendency for assortative mating (persons with similar disorders marrying each other) has been reported repeatedly in affective disorders. It is not known whether this increases the genetic risks, but it does give a peculiar quality to many of the marriages [28]. Among the NIMH inpatients, a majority of bipolar patients get divorced. The divorce often is attributed to signs of illness, usually to the signs of mania. Occasionally, I have been confronted with flat questions: my fiancé is a manic depressive, should I marry him or her; or, my husband or wife is a manic depressive, should we have children? Answering these questions requires great clinical skill and compassion. I recall the regrets of the "well spouses" in a recent questionnaire we gave to a group of married bipolar patients and their normal spouses [29]. One of the questions asked, "If you had known then what you know now, would you have married?" Nine out of 10 patients said "yes," but more than half the spouses said they would not.

References

1   Gershon, E.S.; Bunney, W.E., Jr.; Leckman, J.F.; et al.: The inheritance of affective disorders: a review of data and hypotheses. Behav. Genet. *6:* 227–261 (1976).
2   Mendelwicz, J.; Rainer, J.D.: Adoption study supporting genetic transmission in manic depressive illness. Nature, Lond. *268:* 327–329 (1977).
3   Kety, S.S.: Disorders of the human brain. Scient. Am. *241:* 202–214 (1979).
4   Leonhard, K.: Aufteilung der endogenen Psychosen; 2nd ed. Berlin (1959).
5   Leonhard, K.; Korff, I.; Schulz, H.: Die Temperamente in den Familien der monopolaren und bipolaren phasischen Psychosen. Psychiat. Neurol. *143:* 416 (1962).
6   Nurnberger, J.I., Jr.; Roose, S.P.; Dunner, D.L.; et al.: Unipolar mania: a distinctly clinical entity? Am. J. Psychiat. *136:* 1420–1423 (1979).
7   Gershon, E.S.: The search for genetic markers in affective disorders; in Lipton, DiMascio, Killam, Psychopharmacology: a generation of progress, pp. 1197–1212 (Raven Press, New York 1978).
8   Kupfer, D.J.; Pickar, D.; Himmelhoch, J.M.; et al.: Are there two types of unipolar depression? Archs. gen. Psychiat. *32:* 866–873 (1975).
9   Krauthammer, C.; Klerman, G.L.: Secondary mania: manic syndromes associated with antecedent physical illness or drugs. Archs. gen. Psychiat. *35:* 1333–1339 (1978).
10 Kadrmas, A.; Winokur, G.; Crowe, R.: Postpartum mania. Br. J. Psychiat. *135:* 551–554 (1979).

11 Dunner, D.L.; Gershon, E.S.; Goodwin, F.K.: Heritable factors in the severity of affective illness. Biol. Psychiat. *11:* 31–42 (1976).
12 Gershon, E.S.; Bunney, W.E., Jr.; Goodwin, F.K.; et al.: Catecholamines in affective illness: studies with *L*-dopa and alpha-methyl-para-tyrosine; in Ho, McIsaac, Brain chemistry and mental disease, pp. 135–163 (Plenum Press, New York 1971).
13 Akiskal, H.S.; Rosenthal, R.H.; Rosenthal, T.L.; et al.: Differentiation of primary affective illness from situational, symptomatic and secondary depressions. Archs. gen. Psychiat. *36:* 635–643 (1979).
14 Perris, C.: A study of bipolar (manic-depressive) and unipolar recurrent depressive psychoses. Acta psychiat. neurol. scand. *42:* suppl., p. 194 (1966).
15 Spitzer, R.L.; Endicott, J.; Robins, E.: Research diagnostic criteria (RDC) for a selected group of functional disorders (Pamphlet) (Biometrics Research, New York State Psychiatric Institute 1978).
16 Weissman, M.M.; Myers, J.K.: Affective disorders in a U.S. urban community. Archs. gen. Psychiat. *35:* 1304–1309 (1978).
17 Reich, T.; Andreasen, N.C.: A preliminary analysis of the segregation distributions of the primary affective disorders. Annual Meeting of the American College of Neuropsychopharmacology, San Juan, Puerto Rico 1979.
18 Van Valkenburg, C.; Lowry, M.; Winokur, G.; et al.: Depression spectrum disease versus pure depressive disease. J. nerv. ment. Dis. *165:* 341–347 (1977).
19 Schlesser, M.A.; Winokur, G.; Sherman, B.M.: Genetic subtypes of unipolar primary depressive illness distinguished by hypothalamic-pituitary-adrenal axis activity. Lancet *i:* 739–741 (1979).
20 Gershon, E.S.; Mark, A.; Cohen, M.; et al.: Transmitted factors in the morbid risk of affective disorders: a controlled study. J. psychiat. Res. *12:* 301–317 (1975).
21 McCabe, M.S.: Reactive psychoses. Acta psychiat. scand. *259:* suppl., pp. 1–133 (1975).
22 Mazure, C.; Gershon, E.S.: Blindness and reliability in lifetime psychiatric diagnosis. Archs. gen. Psychiat. *36:* 521–525 (1979).
23 Gershon, E.S.; Bunney, W.E., Jr.: The question of X-linkage in bipolar manic-depressive illness. J. psychiat. Res. *13:* 99–117 (1977).
24 Gershon, E.S.; Goldin, L.R.; Lake, C.R.; et al.: Genetics of plasma dopamine-β-hydroxylase (DBH), erythrocyte catechol-O-methyltransferase (COMT), and platelet monoamine oxidase (MAO) in pedigrees of patients with affective disorders; in Usdin, Sourkes, Youdim, Enzymes and neurotransmitters in mental disease (Wiley, London, in press, 1980).
25 Pandey, G.N.; Dorus, E.; Shaughnessy, R.; et al.: Reduced monamine oxidase activity and vulnerability to psychiatric disorders. Annual Meeting of Biological Psychiatry Society, Chicago 1979.
26 Dorus, E.; Pandey, G.N.; Shaughnessy, R.; et al.: Lithium transport across red cell membrane: a cell membrane abnormality in manic-depressive illness. Science, N.Y. *205:* 932–934 (1979).
27 Targum, S.D.; Gershon, E.S.: Genetic counseling for affective illness; in Belma-

	ker, van Praag, Mania: an evolving concept (Spectrum Publications, New York, in press, 1980).
28	Ablon, S.L.; Davenport, Y.B.; Gershon, E.S.; et al.: The married manic. Am. J. Orthopsychiat. *45:* 854–866 (1975).
29	Targum, S.D.; Dibble, E.D.; Davenport, Y.B.; et al.: The family attitude questionnaire: patients and spouses view bipolar illness. Archs. gen. Psychiat. (in press, 1980).
30	Gershon, E.S.; Hamovit, J.R.: Genetic methods and preventive psychiatry. Prog. Neuro-Psychopharmacol. (in press, 1980).
31	Gershon, E.S.: Genetics of the affective disorders. Hosp. Pract. *14:* 117–122 (1979).

Discussion

Dunner: I would like to comment on the applicability of a genetic model to psychiatry in terms of our studies on life stresses. A genetic model familiar to all of us fits very well into this discussion. I'm referring to sickle cell trait. Sickle cell trait is a genetic disorder that clinically becomes apparent only in the presence of a noxious stress, such as low oxygen tension. Now, applying this sort of model to psychiatric disorders, perhaps we have not been examining the stresses that relate to genetic disposition. Perhaps these stresses have to be specific to interact with the genetic component.

Carroll: I think our research and treatment strategies will be most applicable if the markers we use are closer to the central dysfunction of the illness.

Mendels: To what extent can our present knowledge of genetic factors be used by the clinician in issues of diagnosis or selection of treatment? The data imply that persons with mild depressions have a higher incidence of family history of depression than the control group. To what extent should the clinician be concerned with using family history as part of the diagnostic approach in patients with mild depressions or with somatic symptomatology? To what extent are genetic factors important in selecting appropriate treatment? Does our knowledge on this subject allow us to proceed on this basis at the present time?

Gershon: In terms of treatment choice, genetic factors play a role only in rare instances. For example, when a patient with mild depression has an identical twin with bipolar manic depressive disorder, we assume our patient has the same disease. Therefore, we prescribe lithium although we don't generally treat mild depression with lithium. Other guidelines I use include treating a patient with minor depression as if this illness were much more severe provided the patient has a first-degree relative with severe manic depression.

Mendels: To what extent is history of alcoholism in the family a diagnostic clue to depression?

Winokur: In a Danish adoption study we found that boys born of alcoholic parents but separated at birth (i.e., adopted) were more likely to become alcoholic than boys in a control group. Girls born of alcoholic parents, who lived with their biologic parents, were much more likely to have depression than would be expected by chance. Girls born of alcoholic parents but separated at birth (i.e., adopted) were no more likely to have depression than anyone else in the general population. This gives us some ideas about persons at risk of depression and under what circumstances depression might manifest itself. If it turns out that depression is a genetic illness (manifesting as alcoholism in men and depression in women), then those genetic factors might be relevant in terms of management. I think clinicians can and do use family history in making decisions about treatment.

Dunner: Dr. Frazer, how difficult is it to reconcile the idea that a drug may be an antidepressant although it does not act via the system you outlined?

Frazer: I have no problem with that. Mianserin is a good example of a drug that does not produce beta-adrenergic receptor subsensitivity as measured by DHA binding but, using cyclic AMP as the measure in the limbic forebrain, mianserin does lower noradrenergic responsiveness. What may be important here is development of reduced output. I see no reason to assume that antidepressants work in only one way. Considering the heterogeneity of the condition, it seems quite possible that antidepressants exert their effects through a number of mechanisms. However, since we've shown specific positive results with a number of drugs, I believe that our system has considerable potential in antidepressant screening in preclinical trials.

Maas: I want to emphasize that chronic treatment with drugs has multiple points of entry into multiple points of regulation. Whether a drug does act or not on a biochemical marker does not necessarily reflect the overall integrated function of that drug. While it is comforting to find similar actions among a series of drugs, it does not mean that they will have similar effects in terms of overall functioning of the system. Many mechanisms probably are involved.

Dunner: Many psychiatric residents are being trained to give amphetamines and to choose drug treatment on that basis rather than by looking at the clinical symptomatology of depression. I think they get mixed results. Dr. Maas, can you summarize the status of the amphetamine test?

Maas: I don't think adequate studies have been carried out. The original findings on the relationship between amphetamine response and subsequent treatment response came from a very small sampling of subjects. When we started a relatively large study, many of our patients did not respond to amphetamines at all. Most of these patients had normal MHPG, but that was serendipitous. In answer to your question, I must say that the value of the amphetamine test in clinical practice is not established.

Mendels: Another problem with the studies is the lack of placebo controls. We know that depressed patients in general, especially hospitalized patients, have a significant response to placebo. We have unpublished data showing that some patients receiving placebo demonstrate what appears to be an amphetamine response.

Carroll: How do the type A and type B categories of depressive patients relate to the unipolar and bipolar categories?

Maas: They don't match at this point. I don't have an explanation for it at this time. It seems that *Beckman and Goodwin,* employing a small number of subjects, replicated our original findings. However, they had to exclude bipolar patients to duplicate our results. Of all depressed patients, I think there is general agreement that bipolar depressives have lower urinary MHPG than unipolar patients. Nonetheless, this is the group where prediction of response to imipramine did not hold up.

Carroll: What about the issue of drugs precipitating mania?

Maas: We don't have sufficient knowledge to understand what a drug might be doing in terms of overall functioning of the system, so I cannot answer that question. Based on the current data, I have abandoned the idea of thinking about response to TCA only in terms of blockade of NE reuptake.

Janowsky: Technically, is it possible that a mood response to amphetamine could predict tricyclic response?

Maas: Yes.

Mendels: Before we get caught in the question of whether different kinds of patients respond to different TCAs, let's recall that none of the studies demonstrated that the so-called treatment failures had an adequate therapeutic trial. Given what we know about the metabolic differences of these drugs, the potential importance of plasma and tissue levels, the possible role of hydroxymetabolites, and so on, can we really call any patient a nonresponder unless we apply the best of our current knowledge, measure these variables in a particular patient, and demonstrate certain minimal criteria of treatment exposure? Until that is done, we cannot be sure. Furthermore, it is possible that patients who are drug responders respond to most drugs, not just to one or two, provided they get adequate exposure.

Maas: In terms of plasma level studies, we do need better and larger scale studies. But I think our original data are valid in terms of adequate dosages. Although, in the past, lower doses of TCAs were generally used, our patients received 250–300 mg of imipramine daily. This is the current recommended dosage.

Hartman: In treating depressed patients, I generally prescribe a sedating antidepressant, like amitriptyline, to patients who are very agitated or have difficulty sleeping, and a nonsedating antidepressant to patients who have psychomotor retardation or hypersomnia. I wonder whether your measurements of MHPG levels have anything to do with adrenergic tone in general and whether it correlates with degree of agitation versus retardation?

Maas: Yours is a common practice. However, nothing in the literature suggests that the agitated patient should receive amitriptyline. In fact, new data suggest that the opposite may be true. As for correlating MHPG levels with agitation or retardation, of seven studies conducted only one found that agitation had a significant effect on MHPG levels. However, there was some covariation with stress or anxiety.

Janowsky: Are the multiple effects of tricyclic antidepressants secondary to the blockade of NE reuptake or do they occur for other reasons?

Maas: Many effects are predictable as a function of drug action on reuptake blockade. This includes the change in both pre- and postsynaptic receptor sensitivity. However, the issue becomes complicated. There may be differential sensitivities between postsynaptic receptors and autoreceptors. Therefore, many changes that occur with chronic treatment may occur as a consequence of that chronic treatment with the drugs. I point out that iprindole, for example, does not block reuptake but does have a similar effect on postsynaptic receptor sensitivity as drugs that inhibit NE reuptake. Therefore, many mechanisms are probably involved.

Norepinephrine Neuronal System Functioning and Depression

James W. Maas and Yung Huang

Department of Psychiatry, Yale University School of Medicine, New Haven, Connecticut

In 1968, it was reported that patients who had excellent therapeutic responses to treatment with imipramine or desmethylimipramine (DMI) had low pretreatment urinary values of the major brain metabolite of norepinephrine (NE): 3-methoxy-4-hydroxyphenethyleneglycol (MHPG). Those patients, on the other hand, who were unequivocal nonresponders to these medications had normal or higher than normal urinary MHPG values [1]. The number of subjects in this initial study was small, and, therefore, the investigation was repeated. In the second study, in addition to obtaining measures of MHPG, assays of urinary vanillylmandelic acid, normetanephrine, metanephrine, and NE were carried out. Again, a relation between the pretreatment levels of urinary MHPG and the subsequent response to imipramine was found. This relation was clearly present regardless of whatever measure of change or improvement was used [2]. Finally, no relation between other pretreatment catecholamine metabolites (vanillylmandelic acid, normetanephrine or metanephrine) and the subsequent response to imipramine was found [2].

In another report, *Schildkraut* [3] noted that patients who had normal or greater than normal pretreatment values of urinary MHPG responded well to amitriptyline, whereas a low value for MHPG was associated with a history of failure to respond to amitriptyline. *Beckman and Goodwin* [4] confirmed and extended these findings in patients treated with both amitriptyline and imipramine and who were classified as unequivocal responders or nonresponders to each of the medications. They found that patients who were categorized as unequivocal responders to amitriptyline had higher pretreatment values of urinary MHPG than those who were unequivocal nonresponders to this drug. Conversely, patients with the lower pretreatment urinary MHPG values were unequivocal responders to imipramine, whereas those patients with the higher urinary MHPG values were, again, unequivocal responders to this agent. In these studies, the results emerge most clearly if patients are classified as responders or nonresponders and the intermediate groups are excluded.

Cobbin et al. [5] took these findings, which had been obtained in special research settings, and applied them to a routine clinical situation, i.e., they used MHPG values to determine which type of tricyclic antidepressant should be used. They studied 43 comparison and 35 experimental patients and found that the use of the pretreatment urinary MHPG level as the criterion for drug selection resulted in significantly better clinical results than had been obtained using more traditional selection methods.

About the same time when some of the earlier studies dealing with response to imipramine or DMI and pretreatment MHPG values were being conducted, a separate series of investigations was performed to see whether one could predict efficacy of treatment with imipramine by giving a trial of *d*-amphetamine. The purpose of these studies was to obtain a method whereby one could shortcut the necessity of waiting 3–4 weeks to find out whether a patient would respond to imipramine. In these studies, *d*-amphetamine was given alternatively with placebo, using a double-blind design, and changes in the mood of the patient were noted. Those patients who subsequently had a favorable response to treatment with impramine had a brightening of mood when given *d*-amphetamine, whereas those patients who failed to respond to imipramine did not have an elevation of mood with this drug [6]. Coincident with these results was the finding noted above that there was a relation between pretreatment with MHPG and the subsequent treatment response to imipramine. For this reason, the preamphetamine urines of these patients were assayed for MHPG. It was found that those patients who had an elevation of mood after administration of *d*-amphetamine had lower pretreatment urinary MHPG values than those who did not have a brightening of mood after a trial with *d*-amphetamine [7].

Van Kammen and Murphy [8] also investigated relationships between the therapeutic response to imipramine and changes in activation, depression, and euphoria as induced by an earlier trial with *d*-amphetamine. With inpatients first given *d*-amphetamine and then treated with imipramine, they found significant correlations between *d*-amphetamine-induced changes in activation, euphoria, and depression with the antidepressant effects of imipramine. However, when they administered d-amphetamine to outpatients who had previously failed to respond to a trial with imipramine, similar responses to d-amphetamine were found.

Given these data, it has been suggested that depressed patients may be separated biochemically and pharmacologically into at least two categories [9]: group A consists of patients with a low pretreatment MHPG level, a favorable response to treatment with imipramine or DMI, a brightening of mood after a trial of d-amphetamine, and a failure to respond to amitriptyline; in group B patients are characterized by a normal or high urinary MHPG level, a favorable treatment response to amitriptyline, a lack of mood change during a trial of d-amphetamine, and a failure to respond to imipramine.

Based on acute pharmacologic modes of action of imipramine and amitriptyline [9] as well as on reports which indicate that MHPG production may serve as a marker for the functional activities in CNS neurons [10], it was suggested that the biochemically and pharmacologically defined A type of depression was associated with a disorder, probably central, in the functioning of noradrenergic neuronal systems. The nature of this suggested disorder was not elaborated. However, it was noted that biochemical and pharmacologic characteristics of type A depression were generally consistent with the catecholamine hypothesis of affective disorders, i.e., some depressive states are associated with a deficiency of CNS NE, and some manic states are associated with an excess of this neurotransmitter [11, 12].

Over the past several years, however, a more complete understanding has emerged regarding the mechanisms by which noradrenergic neurons are regulated. Also, some previously unknown pharmacologic effects of chronically administered antidepressant drugs have been elucidated. These newer findings have resulted in important revisions of hypotheses which relate the functioning of NE neuron systems to affective illnesses. In this paper, these newer data and hypotheses which emerge from them will be reviewed. Finally, an attempt will be made to integrate these newer data and hypotheses with the noted biologic characteristics of type A depression to arrive at a hypothesis about the pathophysiology of NE neuronal systems which may occur in this subgroup of depressive disorders.

A brief review of the multiple points at which NE neuron function is regulated, both biochemically and physiologically, and the relevance of this in interpreting the effects of antidepressant drugs on these systems is presented below.

Some of these points of regulation are schematically noted in figure 1 and are listed below with explanatory comments.

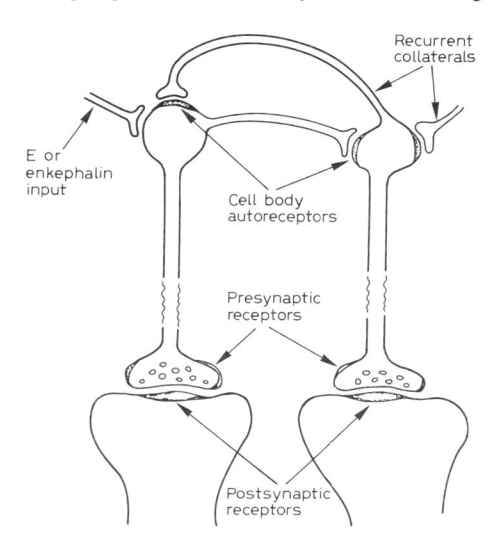

Fig. 1. Schematic view of some regulatory mechanisms which influence the functioning of the *NE neuron-following cell complex*.

Autoreceptors

Presynaptic Autoreceptors
They modulate the quanta of neurotransmitter released per impulse. It is currently thought that presynaptic α_2-receptors function to produce a decrement in NE released per impulse during periods of heightened impulse flow, and an increment in NE released per impulse during periods of decreased impulse flow [13, 14]. There is also evidence suggesting that β-receptors exist in some presynaptic terminals and that, in contrast to α_2-receptors, these β-receptors enhance neurally mediated NE release [14–17].

Cell Body Autoreceptors
These provide a mechanism for self-inhibition of impulse flow, probably via recurrent collaterals, i.e., increased impulse flow in NE neurons is associated with an increased release of NE onto cell body autoreceptors. This results in a decrease in the firing of neurons [18, 19]. As with presynaptic α_2 receptors, this mechanism might also provide a buffering effect on neurotransmitter release during changes in impulse flow.

Synthesis and Degradation of NE

Since the enzyme tyrosine hydroxylase normally is saturated with the amino acid tyrosine at physiologic concentrations, and because the step which is catalyzed by this enzyme (i.e., the conversion of tyrosine to dihydroxyphenylalanine) is rate limiting in the synthesis of NE (fig. 1, 2), the quantity of tyrosine hydroxylase present in the neuron might serve to regulate the amount of NE synthesized [20]. Similarly, upon release, NE is in part metabolized. Consequently, factors which alter the rate of degradation could affect the amount of NE available for either reuptake or interaction with the postsynaptic receptor. For example, as will be noted later, alterations in the amount of available S-adenosylmethionine, a necessary cofactor in the metabolism of NE, might alter the rate of degradation of the neurotransmitter.

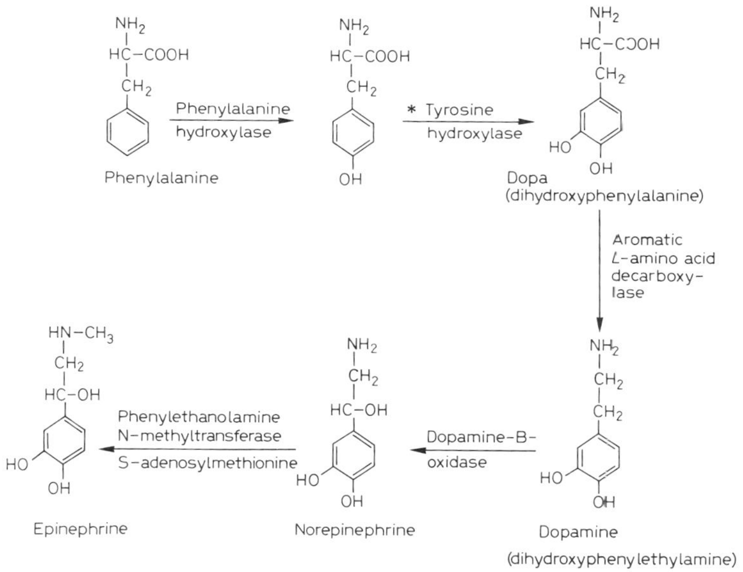

Fig. 2. De novo synthesis of norepinephrine. None of the enzymes in this system is highly specific. Tyrosine hydroxylase (*) is the rate-limiting step in NE synthesis. Inhibition of this enzyme leads to depletion of NE. Hydroxylation of tyrosine to dopa and decarboxylation of dopa to dopamine occurs in the cytoplasm. Dopamine then enters the granules where it is converted to NE. In the adrenal medulla NE leaves the granules, is methylated in the cytoplasm to epinephrine and reenters a different group of intracellular granules where it is stored until release.
(Reprinted by permission from Louis S. Goodman and Alfred Gilman: *The Pharmacological Basis of Therapeutics,* 4th Edition, page 423, Figure 21-5. Copyright 1970, Macmillan Publishing Co., New York.)

The Reuptake Mechanism

The principal means of inactivation of NE is by reuptake [21]. Alterations here also might be expected to alter the amount of NE available to both postsynaptic and autoreceptors. Alterations in this reuptake mechanism, by whatever means, would thus have direct and perhaps opposite effects upon the functioning of NE systems. Thus, blockade of reuptake might yield more NE for interaction with postsynaptic receptors, but it might also increase the amount of NE which interacts with autoreceptors, thereby ultimately reducing the amount of NE released per impulse.

Modulatory Inputs

The locus ceruleus (LC), which contains the cell bodies of origin of approximately 75% of NE neurons in the primate brain [22], receives an extensive enkephalin input [23] as well as inputs from epinephrine neuronal systems [24]. It is possible, although not yet demonstrated, that these input systems provide a method by which activity of NE neuronal systems might be amplified or diminished.

Postsynaptic Receptor Sensitivity

Changes in the sensitivity of the NE receptor on the following postsynaptic cells would be expected to markedly affect the functional efficiency of the presynaptic NE neuron.

For ease of presentation, each of these points of regulation has been described separately. However, this piecemeal description should not obscure the reality that all points of regulation are simultaneously operative and the net activity of the NE neuron-following cell complex is integral to all mechanisms (fig. 3). It also should be emphasized that changes in the biochemistry and functioning of the NE neuron may reflect events in only those neurons and not in the following cell. In most if not all cases, the following cell will utilize a chemically different transmitter. For this reason, measures of biochemical markers of the activity of NE neurons per se during drug treatment will not necessarily yield specific information on the effect of a drug on the functional activity of the NE neuron-following cell complex. This is an important point, albeit obvious, since theories as to the pathophysiology of illness (in this case

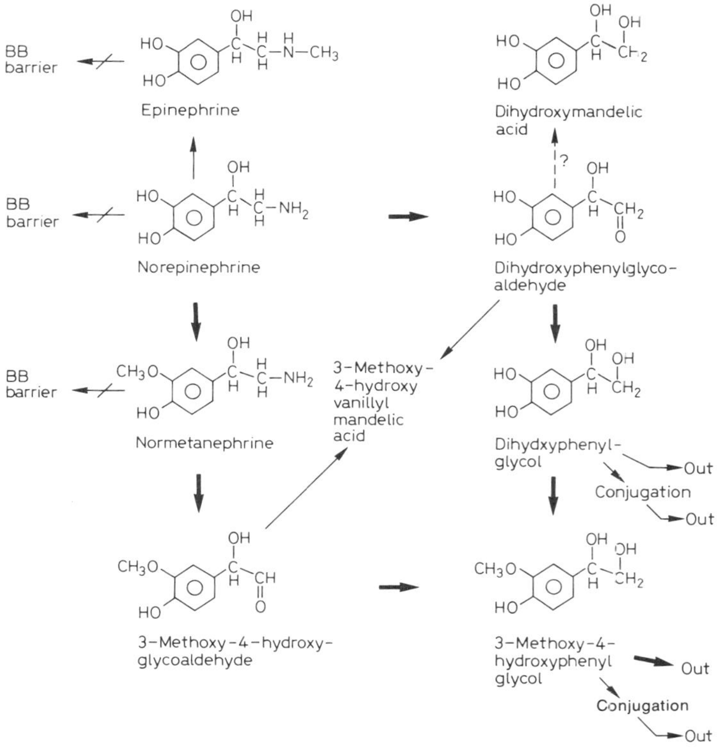

Fig. 3. Metabolism and degradation of norepinephrine. Epinephrine, NE, and normetanephrine cannot cross the blood-brain barrier. Most of the NE that enters the circulation, or is released rapidly from adrenergic fibers, is first methylated via catechol-*o*-methyltransferase to metanephrine or normetanephrine. NE that is released slowly by drugs or by low-frequency nerve impulses probably is deaminated by monoamine oxidase and converted rapidly to 3,4-dihydroxymandelic acid. In either case, most of the metabolite then is converted to 3-methoxy-4-hydroxymandelic acid (VMA), the major metabolite of catecholamines excreted in the urine. In human brain, the aldehyde oxidation products of monoamine oxidase are reduced, resulting in MHPG, the major metabolite of NE in the brain. Varying amounts of these metabolites are conjugated to corresponding sulfates of glucuronides before urinary excretion.
(Reprinted by permission from J. Maas: "Clinical and biochemical heterogenity of depressive disorders," *Annals of Internal Medicine,* Vol. 88, No. 4, pp. 556–563, April 1978.)

depression) are often derived from the effects of pharmacologic agents on the biochemistry and/or functioning of the presynaptic neuron only, rather than from the effects of the drug on the functional activity of the presynaptic neuron-following cell unit. Similarly, information regarding the biochemistry and pharmacology of the postsynaptic receptors alone will not necessarily reflect the integrated functioning of the NE neuron-following cell unit.

Earlier research with the tricyclic antidepressant drugs focused upon the acute effects of these agents in blocking the reuptake of NE and other neurotransmitters. More recent pharmacologic investigations have examined the effect of chronic administration, because therapeutic effects of the tricyclic antidepressants are not seen acutely but only after 2–4 weeks' treatment. Furthermore, research has shifted to examination of the effects of these drugs on regulatory processes (as reviewed above) which may alter the functioning of the NE neuron-following cell unit. Some recent findings on changes that occur with chronic antidepressant drug treatment and the inferred alterations in functional activity are described below.

Synthesis

Chronic treatment with DMI produces a decrement in the amount of tyrosine hydroxylase in the brain [25]. Since this enzyme is the rate-limiting step in the production of NE, it might be expected that chronic treatment with DMI would be associated with decreased synthesis of NE. This expectation is supported by the finding that chronic treatment with DMI produces a small but significant decrease in the endogenous content of NE in the brain [26].

Reuptake

As noted, the original experiments with the tricyclic antidepressants focused on their blockade of the reuptake of neurotransmitters when given acutely. It seemed possible that with chronic treatment this effect might be diminished or lost. However, experimental evidence indicates that even with chronic treatment DMI has potent effects upon this mechanism in NE neurons [26].

3-Methoxy-4-Hydroxyphenethyleneglycol

Since MHPG changes with impulse flow in NE neurons, measurement of this metabolite during chronic treatment with antidepressant drugs has been examined to assess drug effects on the functional activity of NE systems [10]. Results in animals indicate that chronic treatment with imipramine or DMI produces an increase in brain MHPG which could be indicative of increased activity in NE neurons [27, 28]. Interpretation of data from human subjects is more difficult for the following reasons. Chronic treatment with antidepressant drugs which block the reuptake of NE is associated with a decrement in cerebrospinal fluid or urinary MHPG when patients are taken as a group. There is suggestive evidence, however, that the level of MHPG in cerebrospinal fluid or urine may change as a function of the therapeutic response of the patient, i.e., patients who respond well to treatment may have modest increments in MHPG, whereas nonresponders have decrements [29].

Postsynaptic Receptor Sensitivity

It has been found that chronic treatment with DMI, monoamine oxidase inhibitors, and electroshock therapy produces a decrease in the sensitivity of postsynaptic β-noradrenergic receptors [30]. This is due, either totally or in part, to a decrease in the density of these β-adrenergic receptors [31]. These findings have led to the suggestion that antidepressant treatments produce their effects by decreasing postsynaptic receptor sensitivity [30].

NE Degradation

Chronic treatment with imipramine or DMI results in a diminution in the levels of the cofactor S-adenosylmethionine. Since this cofactor is necessary for o-methylation of NE, a major metabolic degradation step (fig. 3), it has been suggested that this effect of chronic treatment with DMI would make more NE available to the postsynaptic receptor [32].

Autoreceptor Sensitivity

Indirect evidence suggests that chronic treatment with DMI produces a decreased sensitivity of autoreceptors on presynaptic membranes and cell bodies [33, 34]. This effect would be expected to produce cell bodies which were less sensitive to self-inhibition, and terminals which were less sensitive to NE overflow; i.e., the postulated net result of chronic administration of the drug would be to produce a hyperactivity of NE neurons.

Basal Firing Rates

The basal firing rate of cell bodies within the LC is decreased with chronic treatment with imipramine or DMI and this effect would be expected to produce a decrease in the functional state of CNS NE neurons [34].

From this review it is apparent that chronic treatment with the antidepressant drugs have a multiplicity of effects and that some of these are expected to be associated with an increase in the functioning of the NE-following cell complex while others are expected to produce a decrease. Depending on how one weighs the results and balances the equation, rather different views of the chronic effects of antidepressant drugs can be developed. This point is illustrated in table I, which lists the findings according to their support for opposing propositions. Viewing these results in this way, it may be seen that by using bits and pieces of pharmacologic or biochemical data to develop a theory regarding the functioning of the NE neuron-following cell complex one might arrive at diametrically opposite hypotheses. Even taking into account all the available biochemical and pharmacologic data, one still cannot infer drug effects in favor of one or the other of the opposing propositions because there is no way to quantitatively weigh the variety of effects produced by the antidepressant drugs.

Table I. Summary of experimental results which support opposing propositions as to the effects of chronic imipramine or DMI administration on CNS NE systems.

Proposition 1 [1]	Proposition 2 [2]
1 Decrease tyrosine hydroxylase	1 Increase MHPG
2 Decrease endogenous brain NE	2 Block reuptake
3 Decrease postsynaptic β-adrenergic receptor sensitivity	3 Decrease S-adenosylmethionine
4 Decrease postsynaptic β-adrenergic receptor density	4 Decrease the sensitivity of α_2-autoreceptors on cell bodies and terminals
5 Decrease basal firing rate of the locus ceruleus	

[1] Antidepressant drugs have the following actions and hence produce a *decrease* in the functional state of CNS NE systems
[2] Antidepressant drugs have the following actions and hence produce an *increase* in the functional state of CNS NE systems
(Reprinted by permission from J. Maas: "Neuron transmitters and depression: Too much, too little or too unstable?" in *Trends in Neuro Sciences.* Copyright 1979, Elsevier/North Holland, Amsterdam.)

The neural projection from NE-containing cells in the LC to the hippocampus has been described in detail with respect to its anatomy [35–38], pharmacology [39–41], and neurophysiology [43, 44].

Activation of the LC, as well as direct application of NE, has been shown to decrease spontaneous activity of a majority of hippocampal cells [43, 44]. Thus, it is possible to study the activity of follower cells by examining those hippocampal cells with a known NE input as determined by a demonstration of inhibition after LC stimulation. Using this LC-hippocampal connection as a test system, it has been found that hippocampal cells inhibited by LC stimulation showed increased firing rates following daily injection for 3 weeks of 5 or 10 mg/kg i.p. of DMI (fig. 4) [45].

The relationship between the length of DMI treatment and the changes in the finding rates of following cells was also examined. In these experiments, it was found that DMI given for 1 day did not alter the baseline activity of LC-responsive hippocampal cells. However, hippocampal activity showed a 20 and a 38% increase after 1 and 2 weeks, respectively, and a statistically significant 89% increase after 3 weeks of the drug treatment (fig. 5). This time course of hippocampal increase is similar to that required to achieve an effect of the drug.

To determine whether the effects on follower cell activity obtained with DMI treatment can be applied to other tricyclic antidepressants, a similar experiment was performed using iprindole. Although similar to DMI in its clinical efficacy, this drug does not alter NE reuptake [46, 47] nor is it a monoamine oxidase inhibitor [46].

A single dose of iprindole, given either intravenously or intraperitoneally, did not alter the firing rate of LC-responsive hippocampal cells. On the other hand, daily intraperitoneal injections for 3 weeks of 10 mg/kg iprindole resulted in a 48% increase in the firing rate of LC-responsive hippocampal cells. Thus, the net effect of chronic iprindole treatment, like that of chronic DMI treatment, is antagonistic to the functioning of the LC-hippocampal system. These findings suggest that the net or integrated effect of the antidepressants DMI or iprindole on the NE neuron-following cell complex is one of suppression, i.e., this measure of the integrated functioning of the NE neuron-following cell complex during chronic treatment with these antidepressant drugs is supportive of proposition 1 (table I).

Whether a similar conclusion can be applied to other noradrenergic systems in the CNS remains to be determined. Recently, *Siggins and Schultz* [48] reported that daily intragastric administration of 50 mg/kg of DMI for 3 days and 30 mg/kg for 7–11 days produces a significant decrease in the firing rate of cerebellar Purkinje cells. The reasons for the difference between this and our findings are not readily apparent. It could be owing to differences in the noradrenergic systems studied or to the different dosages used.

The conclusion that chronic treatment with DMI or iprindole is antagonistic to the functioning of the LC-hippocampal system should hold whether the function of NE neurons is inhibitory or modulatory. Recently, it has been reported that following iontophoretic application of NE the response of cerebellar Purkinje cells to other inputs was decreased less than the spontaneous activity of these cells [49]. Thus, NE may have facilitated the response by increasing the signal-to-noise ratio. If the functioning of NE is indeed modulatory, then an increase in the firing rate of LC-responsive hippocampal cells following chronic drug treatment may lead to a decrease in the signal-to-noise ratio when other inputs are applied to the hippocampus. In this case, the conclusion still holds that chronic antidepressant treatment is antagonistic to the functioning of the LC-hippocampal system.

These neurophysiologic data suggest that chronic treatment with DMI or iprindole results in a situation in which the net or overall functioning of the NE neuron-following cell complex is characterized by an increase in the firing rates of the follower cells. Since the NE input to these following cells is inhibitory, this finding is opposite to that which might have been predicted from earlier experimental results which emphasized the blockade of reuptake or NE. Similarly, using these data to understand the functioning of the NE-following cell systems in patients with depression, one can hypothesize that this illness, at least for some patients, is associated with a decrease in the activity of NE-innervated follower cells in the hippocampus. As before, this hypothesis is not isomorphic with the earlier catecholamine theory of the affective disorders [11, 12]. However, it is consistent with recent reports which have emphasized the effects of chronic antidepressant drug treatment on decreasing the sensitivity of postsynaptic receptors [30] and producing decrements in tyrosine hydroxylase [25]. In short, the results obtained with this neurophysiologic technique raise the possibility that the functioning of the NE neuron-following cell complex in the depressed patient is the opposite of that which was originally suggested.

Given these data from pharmacologic and neurophysiologic studies of animals and the characteristics of type A patients noted earlier (i.e., decreased urinary MHPG, a mood elevation with *d*-amphetamine and a favorable response to imipramine or DMI), what might be the pathophysiology in the NE neuron-following cell complex which is associated with this depressive subgroup? It is suggested that these patients develop a postsynaptic supersensitivity, followed by a compensatory increase in the sensitivity of α_2-autoreceptors on cell bodies and presynaptic terminals, which results in decreased activity in the follower cells. In this model, the compensatory change in the autoreceptors cannot totally correct for the increased postsynaptic receptor sensitivity. In this situation presumably less MHPG would be formed due to (1) the decrement of NE neuronal activity and (2) the decreased NE release which would occur as a result of the supersensitivity of presynaptic and cell body α_2-autoreceptors. It is also expected that a mood elevation might result from d-amphetamine treatment. Imipramine or DMI would produce an increase in the activity of the follower cells (and hence therapeutic response) as a result of inducing a decreased sensitivity in both postsynaptic and presynaptic autoreceptors [30, 31, 33, 34].

Several experimental approaches for testing this hypothesis are available. First, and perhaps most important, drugs which produce an increase in the

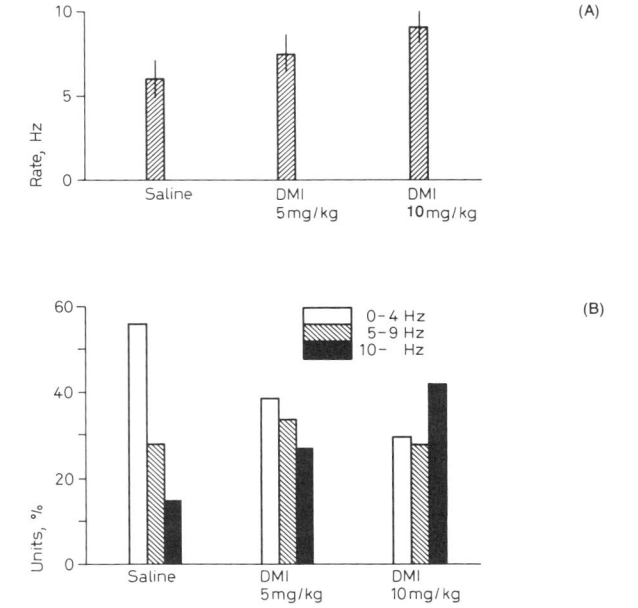

Fig. 4. A Mean firing rates of LC-responsive hippocampal pyramidal cells recorded from different groups of rats. B Percentages of units firing at 0–4.9, 5.0–9.9 or faster Hz. The difference between the saline and the 10 mg/kg DMI groups was significant ($t = 2.03$, d.f. = 68, p. < .05 for A; $\chi^2 = 7.03$, d.f. = 2, p < .05 for B).
(Reprinted by permission from Yung H. Huang: "Chronic desipramine treatment increase activity of noradrenergic postsynaptic cells," *Life Sciences,* Vol. 25, pp. 709–716. Copyright 1979, Pergamon Press, Ltd., New York.)

activity of hippocampal follower cells, by whatever mechanism, should have mood-elevating properties in this defined, type A, subgroup of patients. For example, if the theoretically expected increase in the firing rate of hippocampal follower cells, after small doses of the NE agonist clonidine is demonstrated, this drug should then produce a mood elevation in type A patients. Similarly, if it were demonstrated that NE receptor antagonists produce an increase in the firing rate of follower cells, then these agents should also possess mood-elevating properties. In these experimental approaches, proper attention should be paid to the temporal relationships between the time on drug required to produce a mood change and the length of time on drug required to demonstrate a neurophysiologic effect (fig. 4, 5).

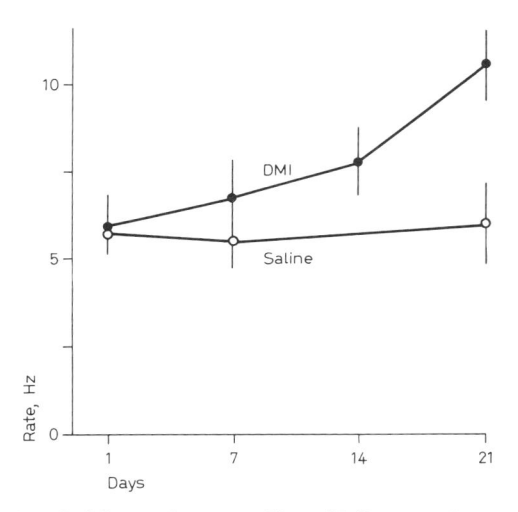

Fig. 5. Mean firing rates (Hz) of LC-responsive hippocampal pyramidal cells plotted against the days of DMI or saline injections. The 21-day DMI group differed significantly from any of the three saline groups. It also differed from all other drug groups except the one treated for 14 days. None of the drug groups treated for less than 21 days differed from the saline groups.

References

1 Maas, J.W.; Fawcett, J.A.; Dekirmenjian, H.: Catecholamine metabolism and the depressive states. Ann. Meet. Am. Psychiat. Ass., Boston 1968.
2 Maas, J.W.; Fawcett, J.A.; Dekirmenjian, H.: Catecholamine metabolism, de-

pressive illness, and drug response. Archs. gen. Psychiat. 26: 252–262 (1972).
3   Schildkraut, J.J.: Norepinephrine metabolites as biochemical criteria for classifying depressive disorders and predicting responses to treatment: preliminary findings. Am. J. Psychiat. 130: 695–698 (1973).
4   Beckman, H.; Goodwin, F.K.: Antidepressant response to tricyclics and urinary MHPG in unipolar patients. Archs. gen. Psychiat. 32: 17–21 (1975).
5   Cobbin, D.M.; Requin-Blow, B.; Williams, L.R.; et al.: Urinary MHPG levels and tricyclic antidepressant drug selection. Archs. gen. Psychiat. 36: 1111–1118 (1979).
6   Fawcett, J.W.; Siomopoulous, V.: Dextroamphetamine response as a possible predictor of improvement with tricyclic therapy in depression. Archs. gen. Psychiat. 25: 247–255 (1971).
7   Fawcett, J.; Maas, J.W.; Dekirmenjian, H.: Depression and MHPG excretion: response to dextroamphetamine and tricyclic antidepressant. Archs. gen. Psychiat. 26: 246–251 (1972).
8   Van Kammen, D.P.; Murphy, D.G.: Prediction of antidepressant response by a one-day d-amphetamine trial. Am. J. Psychiat. 135: 1179–1184 (1978).
9   Maas, J.W.: Biogenic amines and depression. Archs. gen. Psychiat. 32: 1357–1361 (1975).
10 Korf, J.; Aghajanian, G.K.; Roth, R.H.: Stimulation and destruction of the locus coeruleus opposite effects on 3-methoxy-4-hydroxyphenylglycol sulfate levels in the rat cerebral cortex. Eur. J. Pharmacol. 21: 305 (1973).
11 Schildkraut, J.: The catecholamine hypothesis of affective disorders. A review of supporting evidence. Am. J. Psychiat. 122: 508–522 (1965).
12 Bunney, W.E., Jr.; Davis, J.M.: Norepinephrine in depressive reactions. Archs. gen. Psychiat. 13: 483–494 (1965).
13 Starke, K.; Taube, H.D.; Borowski, E.: Presynaptic receptor systems in catecholaminergic transmission. Biochem. Pharmacol. 26: 259–268 (1977).
14 Weiner, N.: Multiple factors regulating the release of norepinephrine consequent to nerve stimulation. Fed. Proc. 38: 2193–2202 (1979).
15 Adler-Graschinsky, E.; Langer, S.Z.: Possible role of a beta-adrenoceptor in the regulation of noradrenaline release by nerve stimulation through a positive feedback mechanism. Br. J. Pharmacol. 53: 43–50 (1975).
16 Farnebo, L.O.; Hamberger, B.: Influence of alpha- and beta-adrenoceptors on the release of noradrenaline from field stimulated atria and cerebral cortex slices. J. Pharm. Pharmacol. 26: 644–646 (1974).
17 Stjarne, L.; Brundin, Y.: Dual adrenoceptor-mediated control of noradrenaline secretion from human vasoconstrictor nerves: facilitation by beta-receptors and inhibition by alpha-receptors. Acta physiol. scand. 94: 139–141 (1975).
18 Aghajanian, G.K.; Cedarbaum, J.M.; Wang, R.Y.: Evidence for norepinephrine-mediated collateral inhibition of locus coeruleus neurons. Brain Res. 136: 570–577 (1977).
19 Cedarbaum, J.M.; Aghajanian, G.K.: Catecholamine receptors on locus coeruleus neurons: pharmacological characterization. Eur. J. Pharmacol. 44: 375–386 (1977).

20 Nagatsu, T.; Levitt, M.; Udenfriend, S.: Tyrosine hydroxylase. J. biol. Chem. 239: 2910–2917 (1964).
21 Whitby, L.G.; Axelrod, J.; Weil-Malherbe, H.: The fate of H^3-norepinephrine in animals. J. Pharmacol. exp. Ther. 132: 193–201 (1961).
22 Huang, Y.; Redmond, E.; Maas, J.M.: Unpublished observations.
23 Pert, C.B.; Kuhar, M.J.; Snyder, S.H.: Autoradiographic localization of the opiate receptor in rat brain. Life Sci. 16: 1849–1854 (1975).
24 Hokfelt, T.; Fuxe, K.; Goldstein, M.; Johansson, O.: Immunohistochemical evidence for the existence of adrenaline neurons in the rat brain. Brain Res. 66: 235–251 (1974).
25 Segal, D.S.; Kuczenski, R.; Mandell, A.J.: Theoretical implications of drug-induced adaptive regulation for a biogenic amine hypothesis of affective disorder. Biol. Psychiat. 9: 147–159 (1974).
26 Schildkraut, J.J.; Winokur, A.; Applegate, C.W.: Norepinephrine turnover and metabolism in rat brain after long-term administration of imipramine. Science 1168: 867–869 (1970).
27 Roffman, M.; Kling, M.A.; Cassens, G.; Orsulak, P.J.; Riegle, T.G.; Schildkraut, J.J.: The effects of accute and chronic administration of tricyclic antidepressants on MHPG-SO_4 in rat brain. Commun. Psychopharmacol. 1: 195–206 (1977).
28 Tang, S.W.; Helmeste, D.M.; Stancer, H.C.: The effect of acute and chronic disipramine and amitriptyline treatment on rat brain total 3-methoxy-4-hydroxyphenethyleneglycol. Archs. Pharmacol. 305: 207–211 (1978).
29 Maas, J.W.: The effect of psychopharmacological agents on CNS amine metabolism in man. Annu. Rev. Pharmacol. Toxicol. 17: 411–424 (1977).
30 Sulser, F.; Vetulani, J.; Mobley, P.L.: Commentary: mode of action of antidepressant drugs. Biochem. Pharmacol. 27: 257–261 (1978).
31 Banerjee, S.P.; Kung, L.S.; Riggi, J.S.; Chanda, S.K.: Development of β-adrenergic receptor subsensitivity by antidepressants. Nature, Lond. 268: 455–456 (1977).
32 Taylor, K.M.; Randall, P.K.: Depletion of S-adenosyl-methionine in mouse brain by antidepressive drugs. J. Pharmacol. exp. Ther. 194: 301–310 (1975).
33 Crews, F.T.; Smith, C.B.: Presynaptic alpha-receptor subsensitivity after long-term antidepressant treatment. Science 202: 322–324 (1978).
34 Svensson, T.H.; Usdin, T.: Feedback inhibition of brain noradrenaline neurons by tricyclic antidepressants: α-receptors mediation. Science 202: 1089–1091 (1978).
35 Kobayashi, R.M.; Palkovits, M.; Kopin, I.S.; Jacobowitz, D.M.: Biochemical mapping of noradrenergic nerves arising from the rat locus coeruleus. Brain Res. 77: 269–280 (1974).
36 Pickel, V.M.; Segal, M.; Bloom, F.E.: A radioautographic study of the efferent pathways of the nucleus locus coeruleus. J. comp. Neurol. 155: 15–42 (1974).
37 Moore, R.Y.: Monoamine neurons innervating the hippocampal formation and septum: organization and response to injury; in Isaacson, Pribram, The hippocampus, pp. 215–238 (Plenum Press, New York 1975).

38 Ungerstedt, U.: Stereotaxic mapping of the monoamine pathways in the rat brain. Acta physiol. scand. *367:* suppl., pp. 1–48 (1971).
39 Korf, J.; Aghajanian, G.K.; Roth, R.H.: Stimulation and destruction of the locus coeruleus: opposite effects on 3-methoxy-4-hydroxyphenylglycol sulfate levels in the rat cerebral cortex. Eur. J. Pharmacol. *21:* 301–310 (1973).
40 Korf, J.; Roth, R.H.; Aghajanian, G.K.: Alterations in turnover and endogenous levels of norepinephrine in cerebral cortex following electrical stimulation and acute axotomy of cerebral noradrenergic pathways. Eur. J. Pharmacol. *23:* 276–282 (1973).
41 Arbuthnott, G.W.; Christie, J.E.; Crow, T.J.; Eccleston, D.; Walter, D.S.: Lesions of the locus coeruleus and noradrenaline metabolism in cerebral cortex. Expl. Neurol. *41:* 411–417 (1973).
42 Walter, D.S.; Eccleston, D.: Increase of noradrenaline metabolism following electrical stimulation of the locus coeruleus. J. Neurochem. *21:* 281–289 (1973).
43 Segal, M.; Bloom, F.E.: The action of norepinephrine in the rat hippocampus. I. Iontophoretic studies. Brain Res. *72:* 79–97 (1974).
44 Segal, M.; Bloom, F.E.: The action of norepinephrine in the rat hippocampus. II. Activation of the input pathway. Brain Res. *72:* 99–114 (1974).
45 Huang, Y.H.: Chronic desipramine treatment increase activity of noradrenergic postsynaptic cells. Life Sci. *25:* 709–716 (1979).
46 Gluckman, M.I.; Baum, T.: The pharmacology of iprindole, a new antidepressant. Psychopharmacologia *15:* 169–185 (1969).
47 Lahti, R.A.; Maickel, R.P.: The tricyclic antidepressants inhibition of norepinephrine uptake as related to potentiation of norepinephrine and clinical efficacy. Biochem. Pharmacol. *20:* 482–486 (1971).
48 Siggins, G.R.; Schultz, J.E.: Chronic treatment with lithium or desipramine alters discharge frequency and norepinephrine responsiveness of cerebellar Purkinje cells. Proc. natln. Acad. Sci. USA *76:* 5987–5991 (1979).
49 Woodward, D.J.; Moises, H.C.; Waterhouse, B.D.; Hoffer, B.J.; Freedman, R.: Modulatory actions of norepinephrine in the central nervous system. Fed. Proc. *38:* 2109–2116 (1979).

Serotonergic Function and Depression

Jay D. Amsterdam and Joseph Mendels

The Fairmount Institute; University of Pennsylvania,
Philadelphia, Pennsylvania

Synthesis of Serotonin and Related Compounds

The indolealkylamines (especially serotonin [5-hydroxytryptamine, 5-HT]) have been implicated in the etiology of endogenous depression. Serotonin is synthesized from the precursor amino acid, tryptophan, in specific neurons located in discrete brain areas. Tryptophan is absorbed through the gut into the bloodstream and, via an active transport system, crosses the blood-brain barrier and enters the central nervous system (CNS) [1]. This transport system is not specific for tryptophan, and amino acids such as phenylalanine and methionine compete for entry sites. A diet deficient in tryptophan eventually leads to decreased serotonin production in the CNS. Similarly, an increased concentration of competing amino acids may lead to decreased tryptophan uptake and diminished serotonin production in the CNS [1].

The cell bodies of most serotonergic neurons are located in the raphe nuclei of the brain stem and mesencephalon. From there, major neuronal pathways project to the forebrain via fibers passing through the median forebrain bundle while other fibers lead into the spinal cord [2].

After uptake into the cells, tryptophan is hydroxylated to 5-hydroxytryptophan, followed by decarboxylation via aromatic acid decarboxylase. Tryptophan-hydroxylase is the rate-limiting enzyme in the synthetic pathway and may, in turn, be regulated by intraneuronal levels of serotonin [3].

Serotonin is also synthesized in cells of the pineal gland which contain a 50 times higher concentration of serotonin per gram of tissue than brain tissue [1]. In addition, pinealocytes contain enzymes for the metabolism of serotonin to melatonin, a hormone that acts as a neural transducer which, among its other actions, modifies the release of pituitary hormones and affects sexual maturation and behavior. The conversion of serotonin to melatonin is controlled by a complex neural pathway dependent on environmental light and mediated, through β-adrenergic receptors, on the pineal cells [4].

Over the last two decades, biochemical and clinical studies have indicated that affective illness may be associated with a functional deficiency of serotonin at certain brain sites. This argument has been strengthened by the fact that some antidepressants increase serotonin levels by inhibiting reuptake into the presynaptic nerve ending; furthermore, it suggests that the clinical effect of these drugs may be due to their increasing the available amine concentration at postsynaptic receptor sites. The evidence for these hypotheses has been reviewed elsewhere [5]. Recent theories concerning possible alterations in serotonin metabolism, receptor sensitivity, and alterations in diurnal rhythms will be presented in this paper.

Measurement of Indole Compounds in Urine and Blood

Investigators have carried out several urine and blood measurements of serotonin activity. The results of these studies, measuring in depressed patients urinary excretion of the serotonin metabolite, 5-hydroxyindoleacetic acid (5-HIAA), are conflicting. Thus, *Garfinkel* et al. [6] found no differences in 24-hour urinary 5-HIAA concentrations between 8 bipolar depressed patients and 10 normal controls. Other investigators, however, have reported elevated urinary 5-HIAA in some patients with depression [7]. In a recent study evaluating the fate of [^{14}C]-*L*-tryptophan metabolism in depressed patients, *Coppen* et al. [8] measured [^{14}C]-5-HIAA excretion in urine of depressed patients and healthy volunteers and reported that no differences were found. It must be noted that data concerning the urinary excretion of 5-HIAA are probably of limited value as far as brain serotonin turnover is concerned. There are reports of diminished concentration of serotonin in platelets [9] and in serum in depressed patients compared with controls or with patients recovered from a depression [10]. These studies must also be interpreted with caution since serotonin does not appear to cross the blood-brain barrier, and serum or platelet measurements of serotonin are unlikely to reflect CNS indoleamine metabolism. The rate of CNS serotonin synthesis is partly dependent on blood levels of tryptophan. Measurement of this precursor might, therefore, be of interest. Early studies by *Coppen* et al. [11] showed that free plasma tryptophan concentrations (i.e., not bound to plasma protein) were diminished in a group of endogenously depressed women as compared with age-matched healthy volunteers. These levels increased when the patients recovered. Other investigators confirmed these findings in postpartum depressed women [12] and in patients with either unipolar or bipolar depression [13]. However, while some investigators found no difference in plasma tryptophan concentrations between unipolar or bipolar depressed patients and controls [14, 15], one group reported an increased concentration of free plasma tryptophan in a diagnostically mixed group of depressed patients [16]. Determining the significance of these claims presents many problems. For example, different research methodologies (e.g., diet and fasting time before blood sampling), diagnosis, and normal variations in tryptophan metabolism during different phases of the menstrual cycle may confound the results.

Furthermore, some investigators measured total (bound + unbound) tryptophan plasma levels while others evaluated free (unbound) tryptophan plasma levels. Under physiologic conditions, only the free fraction crosses the blood-brain barrier, although total plasma tryptophan provides a close estimate of the amount of amino acid actually available to the CNS [17]. There is also the complex competition between tryptophan and other neutral amino acids for transport across the blood-brain barrier, and this variation in the relative concentrations of these other amino acids can affect the amount of tryptophan entering the CNS. It has furthermore been suggested that an abnormality in the transport system for tryptophan may be important in the genesis of depression [18]. Conceivably, this might be part of a series of changes in transport systems for electrolytes and amino acids [19].

Measurement of Indole Compounds in CNS

While it is not possible to measure central serotonergic function directly in depressed patients, a number of studies report on the concentrations of tryptophan and 5-HIAA in lumbar spinal fluid of patients and controls.

Preliminary studies report diminished lumbar CSF tryptophan concentrations in both unipolar and bipolar depressed patients compared with controls [20], but it is unclear whether lumbar CSF tryptophan concentrations reflect tryptophan brain levels. Some [20–22], but not all [23], investigators have found a reduced 5-HIAA concentration in lumbar spinal fluid in untreated depressed patients compared with controls as well as in manic patients. It has been suggested that psychotic depressives are more likely to have reduced levels of 5-HIAA in CSF than patients with neurotic depression [20, 22]. These patients may also have less delta wave (slow wave) sleep. This is partly controlled by serotonin. Factors such as physical activity, diet, previous medication, sex, age, and duration of illness may all affect these measurements, making it difficult to interpret their significance. Furthermore, studies have shown that there is a gradient in the CSF 5-HIAA concentration from rostral to caudal areas, and that lumbar spinal fluid measurements may not adequately reflect brain concentrations.

The probenecid technique (probenecid inhibits active transport of 5-HIAA out of the CNS) permits the measurement of the rate of serotonin synthesis and turnover [23]. Thus, accumulation of 5-HIAA in the CSF, after probenecid loading, gives information on the rate of serotonin turnover in the CNS. Several investigators have observed a diminished accumulation of 5-HIAA in some depressed [24] and manic patients [23].

In summary, measurement of urinary, plasma, and CSF tryptophan, serotonin, and probenecid-induced CSF 5-HIAA accumulation have produced conflicting results. More controlled studies with larger numbers of well-diagnosed patients will have to be carried out.

Amine Metabolites and Clinical Response

Several investigators have correlated the concentrations of amine metabolites with clinical responses to particular tricyclics in an attempt to identify subtypes of depression. A biochemical classification of depression has been proposed, based on amine metabolite concentration with treatment response. One group (serotonin deficient) is reported to have normal urinary 3-methoxy-4-hydroxyphenylglycol concentrations (MHPG, the main metabolite of brain norepinephrine), and to respond to amitriptyline; or to have reduced CSF levels of 5-HIAA, and to respond to the new antidepressant chlorimipramine. Amitriptyline and chlorimipramine may be more potent reuptake-inhibitors of serotonin than other tricyclics. These patients are said to have a poor response to the tricyclics which exert their main effect on norepinephrine reuptake, such as imipramine or nortriptyline. This group of patients contrasts with those thought to be norepinephrine deficient, who have low concentrations of MHPG in urine or spinal fluid, and who do respond to imipramine or to nortriptyline [25, 26].

It is of interest to note the report by *Glassman* et al. [27], that delusional depressives do not respond to imipramine, and to speculate that such patients may have a serotonin deficiency. It remains to be seen whether they do respond to a drug such as chlorimipramine.

These studies are potentially important, but do require extension and confirmation, e.g., measurements of both MHPG and 5-HIAA in the same patient.

It cannot be assumed, therefore, that a patient with a reduced level of 5-HIAA necessarily has a normal or high concentrations of MHPG, and, therefore, has a serotonergic depression.

Serotonin Precursor Studies

Burns and Mendels [28] describe six prerequisites for the proper interpretation and success of any precursor study [28]: (1) the indole precursor must be readily absorbed after oral administration; (2) it must pass freely across the blood-brain barrier; (3) it must attain adequate CNS levels and physiologic distribution in the brain; (4) enzymes must be present intraneuronally for conversion of the precursor into serotonin; (5) the precursor must not alter the activity of other neurotransmitter systems; and (6) the newly synthesized serotonin must be released physiologically from the presynaptic nerve ending. Although these criteria have not been met for all precursors of serotonin, clinical studies have demonstrated beneficial effects after treatment with some serotonin precursors.

After oral administration of *L*-tryptophan, both free and protein-bound plasma tryptophan levels increase rapidly [29], and the free fraction is actively transported into the CNS. It is hypothesized that increased CNS levels of tryptophan may stimulate serotonin synthesis and reverse the depressive episode. *Broadhurst* [30] administered tryptophan (6 g daily) to 36 chronically relapsing, depressed patients and reported improvement in 28. Recurrence of depressive episodes occurred when tryptophan was discontinued. *Moller* et al. [31] gave *L*-tryptophan (100–200 mg/kg/day) to a group of bipolar depressed patients with plasma levels of neutral amino acids and obtained favorable results. These investigators suggest that a subgroup of depressed patients exists who suffer a dysfunction of the active transport system for tryptophan across the blood-brain barrier, and that such patients might respond to *L*-tryptophan treatment. Others have not confirmed these findings [32].

Plasma tryptophan stimulates hepatic tryptophan pyrrolase, a liver enzyme which rapidly metabolizes *L*-tryptophan. Drugs such as allopurinal and nicotinamide inhibit liver pyrrolase, increasing plasma-free tryptophan available to the CNS [33, 34]. *Shopsin* [35] treated 8 endogenously depressed patients with 4–6 g of tryptophan daily, plus 100–200 mg allopurinal, and reported improvement in 5 patients. *Chouinard* et al. [36] reported that the combination of 6 g of *L*-tryptophan plus 1–5 g of nicotinamide resulted in partial remission of primary depression. It is difficult to determine the true efficacy of *L*-tryptophan in open trials, either alone or in combination with a pyrrolase inhibitor.

Comparisons of L-tryptophan with electroconvulsive therapy (ECT) have yielded conflicting results [30, 37]. Recent double-blind trials comparing L-tryptophan with imipramine showed that both drugs were equally effective [38, 39]. *Herrington* et al. [40] compared 8 g of L-tryptophan with 150 mg of amitriptyline, daily, in depressed patients. There was no difference in response between groups, but the L-tryptophan-treated patients had fewer relapses after a 6-month follow-up, and the investigators speculated that L-tryptophan may also have prophylactic effects.

While it appears that L-tryptophan may be as effective as tricyclic antidepressants, some investigators have questioned the superiority of tricyclic antidepressants over placebo [41]. Therefore, the results of studies comparing L-tryptophan with tricyclic antidepressants should be interpreted cautiously.

Several investigators have used L-tryptophan combined with tricyclic antidepressants. Theoretically, L-tryptophan enhances the synthesis of presynaptic serotonin concentrations, while tricyclics inhibit the reuptake of newly released neurotransmitter, making it more available at the postsynaptic receptor. In two double-blind studies, the combination of L-tryptophan plus tricyclic antidepressants was not superior to treatment with either imipramine [42] or amitriptyline [43] alone. In another study, L-tryptophan appeared to enhance the antidepressant effect of chlorimipramine [44]; however, this could not be confirmed in a further investigation [45].

L-Tryptophan plus MAOI was compared with MAOI alone in two studies, and the combination was found to be superior [42, 43]. Although, in one study, drowsiness was reported frequently [42], the combined therapy was well tolerated in the other [46]. L-Tryptophan has been reported to be effective in the treatment of mania [47]. However, it may be the sedative-hypnotic effects which account for the decrease in psychomotor agitation and improvement of symptoms. For a more complete review of the serotonin system in the treatment of mania, see *Anath* [48].

The immediate precursor of serotonin, 5-hydroxytryptophan (5-HTP) (fig. 1), has been used in clinical studies both alone and in combination with other antidepressants. In a placebo-controlled, double-blind trial, *Van Praag and Korf* [49] reported that up to 3 g of 5-HTP was effective in 3 out of 5 depressed patients who were characterized as having low postprobenecid CSF levels of 5-HIAA. In another study, *Fugiwara and Otsuki* [50] also reported improvement with 5-HTP treatment in some depressed patients characterized by low CSF concentrations of 5-HIAA. The combination of chlorimipramine plus 5-HTP in chronically depressed patients has been reported to be effective in one study [51]. Studies using 5-HTP plus MAOI yield conflicting results [52, 53], as

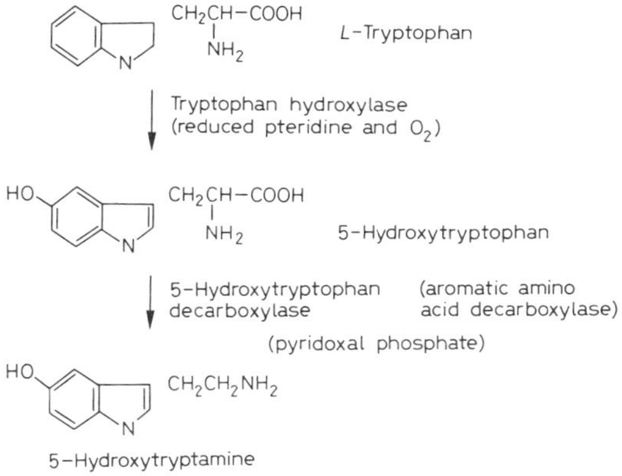

Fig. 1. Biosynthesis of 5-hydroxytryptamine.

have investigations combining 5-HTP with a peripheral decarboxylase inhibitor [54].

In summary, tryptophan-loading studies yield conflicting results as do reports comparing tryptophan with ECT and with tricyclic antidepressants. However, tryptophan may enhance the antidepressant effect of chlorimipramine. Tryptophan plus MAOI was found effective in the treatment of some depressed patients. As a whole, studies using 5-HTP alone or combined with other antidepressants are, at best, equivocal. However, *Van Praag* et al. [49] suggest that there may be a subgroup of depressed patients with low CSF concentrations of 5-HIAA after probenecid, who respond favorably to 5-HTP.

Postmortem Studies

Results from early studies, measuring serotonin levels in the brains of suicide victims, were conflicting [55, 56]. In more recent investigations, *Lloyd* et al. [57] measured serotonin in discrete brain areas of patients who had committed suicide and controls; they found diminished serotonin concentrations in two out of six serotonin-containing raphe nuclei in the brain stem of suicide victims. These studies must be interpreted with caution as many unresolved variables have to be considered: the effects of drugs ingested before death, alterations in serotonin turnover after death, and differences in the patient populations studied.

In a recent combined prospective and retrospective study, *Asberg* et al. [58] measured CSF 5-HIAA concentrations in 68 depressed patients and found that attempted suicide occurred significantly more often among patients with low CSF concentrations of 5-HIAA. These patients also used more violent methods and succeeded more frequently than depressed patients with normal CSF concentrations of 5-HIAA. The authors suggested that 5-HIAA may serve as a predictor for suicidal behavior.

Altered Serotonergic Receptor Sensitivity

Recent studies have focused on possible alterations in neuronal receptor sensitivity as a cause of some affective disorders. One recent review [59] suggests that receptor supersensitivity and/or subsensitivity might explain how environmental or intrapsychic stress could precipitate an affective episode, or the mechanism by which tricyclic antidepressants precipitate mania in some patients with bipolar depression. The authors believe that this might explain the endogenous mechanism which controls the onset and termination (or switch process) of an affective episode. During the depressive phase of illness, a postsynaptic receptor supersensitivity develops with diminished presynaptic release of monoamines. Mania might result from a small but sudden increase in the release of presynaptic serotonin, the effect of which is amplified by the supersensitive postsynaptic receptor. As presynaptic serotonin continues to be released, a subsensitivity develops postsynaptically. A model for serotonergic supersensitivity in laboratory animals has recently been developed. Pretreatment with parachlorophenylalanine (PCPA—an inhibitor of tryptophan hydroxylase) results in animal behavior suggestive of depression, as well as in increased postsynaptic receptor affinity for [^{3}H]-serotonin binding [60].

Savage et al. [67] pretreated rats with types A and B monoamine oxidase inhibitors (MAOI) and measured [^{3}H]-serotonin binding in brain neocortex after 1 day of acute treatment or after 4 or 16 days of chronic treatment. Type A-MAOI significantly increased serotonin concentration and decreased [^{3}H]-serotonin binding at 4 and 16 days. Results from other studies are conflicting [62], and more research is needed to determine a relationship between altered serotonin receptor sensitivity and affective illness.

Neuroendocrine Studies

Recent findings in neuroendocrinology are contributing to the understanding of serotonergic function in depression. *Sachar* et al. [63] described a blunted growth hormone response after insulin-induced hypoglycemia (ITT) in postmenopausal depressed women. Similar growth hormone blunting with ITT has been reported after administration of the serotonin antagonists, cyproheptadine and methysergide [64]. However, the CNS control of growth hormone release is complex, involving many neurotransmitter systems in addition to serotonin. Our preliminary laboratory findings of functional changes in the hypothalamic-pituitary-gonadal axis show baseline follicle-stimulating hormone (FSH) levels significantly higher in postmenopausal depressed women than in a healthy age-matched control group [unpublished data]. Animal data suggest that serotonin exerts a central inhibitory effect on lutenizing hormone (LH) and FSH release [65]. It is possible that the elevated FSH observed in the postmenopausal, depressed women may reflect dysinhibition of the central serotonergic input to the hypothalamic-pituitary-gonadal axis.

Several investigators have observed blunted thyrotropin (TSH) and prolactin release after thyrotropin-releasing hormone (TRH) infusion in approximately 25% of endogenously depressed patients [66, 69]. There is evidence that serotonin may have a stimulatory input for prolactin release as well as for normal phasic release of TSH [68]; moreover, alterations in the indoleamine input to the hypothalamus may contribute to the blunted TSH response, which seems to normalize with clinical remission.

The hypothalamic-pituitary-adrenal (HPA) axis also shows dysinhibition in about 50% of patients with endogenous depression [69]. Resting glucocorticoid levels are elevated [70] and the normal circadian cortisol pattern is obliterated [70]. This is similar to the observation made in centrencephalic Cushing's disease. In addition, the HPA axis shows abnormal early escape from dexamethasone suppression [69, 71, 72] which normalized with clinical improvement [69, 72]. Evidence for serotonin regulation of the HPA axis, whether stimulatory or inhibitory, remains controversial [73]. In animals, interruption of the normal diurnal cortisol rhythm can be induced by a lesion in the serotonin-containing raphe nuclei [73]. A recent clinical investigation showed that tryptophan administration improved the abnormal dexamethasone suppression test in some patients with endogenous depression [72].

Pineal Gland, Circadian Rhythms, and Serotonin Function

Serotonin is synthesized in the pineal gland where it is present in large amounts [1], and is the precursor indole for melatonin. The concentrations of both substances display a circadian rhythm mediated by environmental light through β-noradrenergic receptors on the pineal cells [4].

Melatonin administration has been shown to increase central serotonin levels, suggesting that melatonin might serve as an effective antidepressant in some depressed patients [74]. Clinical studies have demonstrated that baseline plasma and CSF melatonin levels are similar in depressed patients and normal controls. Melatonin administered therapeutically to a group of depressed patients worsened their symptoms, some becoming psychotic [75]. Further studies are needed to determine how melatonin and serotonin interact in depressive illness.

Many depressed patients exhibit diminished stage IV deep sleep and show abnormalities in rapid eye movement (REM) latency [76]. These sleep phennomena are mediated partly through serotonergic neuronal pathways and are entrained in a circadian pattern. It appears that some depressed patients may have an underlying desynchronization of circadian rhythms which may affect serotonin metabolism, melatonin production, and sleep phases [77]. Tricyclic antidepressants advance circadian rhythms and increase cycling time in manic-depressive patients [78]. Lithium carbonate, which interacts with serotonin receptors in the brain, lengthens endogenous rhythms and decreases the severity of manic-depressive episodes [79]. It is tempting to hypothesize that both drugs alter circadian patterns and clinical state by modulating central serotonergic neurotransmission.

Conclusion

Serotonin plays a complex role in the regulation of central neuroendocrine, circadian, and behavioral changes. Functional alteration of serotonin metabolism at specific brain sites may play a role in the development of at least some types of depression. Further studies are necessary to delineate how altered serotonergic regulation in the CNS contributes to depression, whether by depletion of serotonin concentration, by altered serotonin receptor sensitivity, or by another as yet undetermined mechanism.

References

1 Cooper, J.R.; Bloom, F.E.; Roth, R.H.: Serotonin (5HT); in The biochemical basis of neuropharmacology, pp. 177–182 (Oxford University Press, New York 1974).
2 Fuxe, K.: Evidence for the existence of monoamine neurons in the CNS. IV. Distribution of monoamine nerve terminals in the CNS. Acta. physiol. scand. *64:* suppl. 247, pp. 39–85 (1965).

3   Macon, J.B.; Sokoloff, L.; Glowinski, J.: Feedback control of rat brain 5-hydroxytryptamine synthesis. J. Neurochem. *18:* 323–331 (1971).
4   Axelrod, J.: The pineal gland. A neurochemical transducer. Chemical signals from nerves regulate synthesis of melatonin and convey information about internal clocks. Science, N.Y. *184:* 1341–1348 (1974).
5   Davis, J.M.: Theories of biological etiology of affective disorders; in Pfeiffer, Snythies, International review of neurobiology (Academic Press, New York 1979).
6   Garfinkel, P.E.; Warsh, J.J.; Stancer, H.C.; Godse, D.D.: The evaluation of CNS monoamine metabolism in bipolar affective disorder using a peripheral decarboxylase inhibitor. Archs. gen. Psychiat. *34:* 735–739 (1977).
7   Tissot, R.: Monoamines y sindromes maniacode presivas. Neurol. Neurocir. Psquiats. *7:* 53–66 (1966).
8   Coppen, A.; Brooksbank, B.W.L.; Eccleston, E.; White, S.C.: Tryptophan metabolism in depressive illness. Psychol. Med. *45:* 164–173 (1974).
9   Shaw, D.M.; MacSweeney, D.A.; Woolcock, N.; Beven-Jones, A.B.: Uptake and release of ^{14}C-5-hydroxytryptamine by platelets in affective illness. J. Neurol. Neurosurg. Psychiat. *34:* 224–225 (1971).
10 Sarai, K.; Kayamo, M.: The level and diurnal rhythm of serum serotonin in manic-depressive patients. Folia psychiat. neurol. jap. *22:* 271–281 (1968).
11 Coppen, A.; Eccleston, E.G.; Peet, M.: Total and free tryptophan concentrations in the plasma of depressive patients. Lancet *ii:* 60–63 (1973).
12 Stein, G.; Milton, F.; Bebbington, P.; Wood, K.; Coppen, A.: Relationship between mood disturbances and free and total plasma tryptophan in post-partum women. Br. med. J. *ii:* 457 (1976).
13 Nakaya, K.: Serum free tryptophan concentration—the results on the brain serotonin metabolism and its relationship to the mental diseases. Psychiatria Neurol. jap. *78:* 119–132 (1976).
14 Garfinkel, P.E.; Warsh, J.J.; Stances, H.C.; Sibony, D.: Total and free plasma tryptophan levels in patients with affective disorders. Effects of a peripheral decarboxylase inhibitor. Archs. gen. Psychiat. *33:* 1462–1466 (1976).
15 Wirz-Justice, A.; Puhringer, W.; Hole, G.; Menzi, R.: Monoamine oxidase and free tryptophan in human plasma: normal variations and their implications for biochemical research in affective disorders. Pharmakopsychiatry *8:* 310–317 (1975).
16 Niskanen, P.; Huttunen, M.; Tamminen, T.; Jaakelainen, J.: The daily rhythm of plasma tryptophan and tyrosine in depression. Br. J. Psychiat. *128:* 67–73 (1976).
17 Wurtman, R.J.; Pardridge, W.M.: Circulating tryptophan, brain tryptophan, and psychiatric disease. J. neural Transm. *15:* suppl., pp. 227–236 (1979).
18 Moller, S.E.; Amdisen, A.: Plasma neutral amino acids in mania and depression: variations during acute and prolonged treatment with *L*-tryptophan. Biol. Psychiat. *14:* 131–139 (1979).
19 Mendels, J.; Frazer, A.; Carroll, B.: Growth hormone response in depression. Am. J. Psychiat. *131:* 1154–1155 (1974).
20 Coppen, A.; Brooksbank, B.W.L.; Peet, M.: Tryptophan concentration in the cerebrospinal fluid of depressive patients. Lancet *i:* 1393 (1976).

21 Coppen, A.; Prange, A.J.; Whybrow, P.C.; Noguera, R.: Abnormalities of indoleamines in affective disorders. Archs. gen. Psychiat. *26:* 474–478 (1972).
22 Mendels, J.; Frazer, A.; Fitzgerald, R.G.; Ramsey, T.A.; Stokes, J.W.: Biogenic amine metabolism in the cerebrospinal fluid of depressed and manic patients. Science, N.Y. *175:* 1380–1382 (1972).
23 Goodwin, F.K.; Post, R.M.; Dunner, D.L.; Gordon, E.K.: Cerebrospinal fluid amine metabolites in affective illness: the probenecid technique. Am. J. Psychiat. *130:* 73–79 (1973).
24 Van Praag, H.M.; Korf, J.; Puite, J.: 5-Hydroxyindole-acetic acid levels in the cerebrospinal fluid of depressive patients treated with probenecid. Nature, Lond. *225:* 1259–1260 (1970).
25 Maas, J.W.: Biogenic amines and depression. Biochemical and pharmacological separation of two types of depression. Archs. gen. Psychiat. *32:* 1357–1361 (1975).
26 Asberg, M.; Thoren, P.; Traskman, L.: "Serotonin depression." A biochemical subgroup within the affective disorders? Science, N.Y. *191:* 478–480 (1976).
27 Glassman, A.; Kantor, S.; Shostak, M.: Depression, delusions and drug response. Am. J. Psychiat. *132:* 716–719 (1975).
28 Burns, D.D.; Mendels, J.: Serotonin and affective disorders; in Essman, Valzelli, Current development in psychopharmacology, pp. 293–359 (SP Medical and Scientific Books, New York 1979).
29 Greenwood, M.H.; Lader, M.H.; Kahtamenenin, B.D.; Curzon, G.: The acute effects of oral(−)–tryptophan in human subjects. Br. J. clin. Pharmacol. *2:* 165–172 (1975).
30 Broadhurst, A.D.: *L*-Tryptophan vs. ECT. Lancet *i:* 1392–1393 (1970).
31 Moller, S.E.; Kirk, L.; Fremming, K.H.: Plasma amino acid as an index for subgroups in manic depressive psychosis: correlation to effect of tryptophan. Psychopharmacology *49:* 205–213 (1976).
32 Mendels, J.; Stinnett, J.; Burns, D.; Frazer, A.: Amine precursors and depression. Archs. gen. Psychiat. *32:* 22–28 (1975).
33 Chouinard, G.; Young, S.N.; Annable, L.; Sourkes, T.L.: Tryptophan-nicotinamide combination in depression. Lancet *i:* 249 (1977).
34 Badawy, A.A.; Evans, M.: The mechanism of inhibition of rat liver tryptophan pyrrolase activity by 4-hydroxypyrazolo-(3,4-d)-pyrimidine (allopurinol). Biochem. J. *133:* 585–591 (1973).
35 Shopsin, B.: Enhancement of the antidepressant response of *L*-tryptophan by a liver pyrrolase inhibitor: a rational treatment approach. Neuropsychobiology *4:* 188–192 (1978).
36 Chouinard, G.; Young, S.N.; Annable, L.; Sourkes, T.L.; Kiriakos, R.F.: Tryptophan-nicotinamide combination in the treatment of newly admitted depressed patients. Commun. Psychopharmacol. *2:* 311–318 (1978).
37 Herrington, R.N.; Bruce, A.; Johnson, C.; Lader, M.H.: Comparative trial of *L*-tryptophan and ECT in severe depressive illness. Lancet *ii:* 731–734 (1974).
38 Coppen, A.; Whybrow, P.C.; Noguera, R.; Maggs, R.; Prange, A.J., Jr.: The comparative antidepressant value of *L*-tryptophan and imipramine with and without attempted potentiation by liothyronine. Archs. gen. Psychiat. *26:* 234–241 (1972).

39 Rao, B.; Broadhurst, A.D.: Tryptophan and depression. Br. med. J. *i:* 460 (1976).
40 Herrington, R.N.; Bruce, A.; Johnstone, E.C.; Lader, M.H.: Comparative trial of *L*-tryptophan and amitriptyline in depressive illness. Psychol. Med. *6:* 673–678 (1976).
41 Carroll, B.J.; Mowbray, R.M.; Davies, B.: *L*-Tryptophan in depression. Lancet *i:* 1228 (1970).
42 Pare, C.M.B.: Potentiation of monoamine-oxidase inhibitors by tryptophan. Lancet *ii:* 527–528 (1963).
43 Lopez-Ibor, A.J.; Gutierrez, J.L.A.; Inglesias, M.L.M.: Tryptophan and amitriptyline in the treatment of depression. Int. Pharmacopsychiat. *8:* 145–151 (1973).
44 Walender, J.; Skott, A.; Carlsson, A.; Nagy, A.; Roos, B-E.: Potentiation of antidepressant action of clorimipramine. Archs. gen. Psychiat. *33:* 1384–1389 (1976).
45 Shaw, D.M.; Johnson, A.L.; MacSweeney, D.A.: Tricyclic antidepressant and tryptophan in unipolar affective disorder. Lancet *ii:* 1245 (1972).
46 Gutierrez, J.L.A.; Lopez-Ibor, A.J.J.: Tryptophan and an MAOI (Nialamide) in the treatment of depression. Int. Pharmacopsychiat. *6:* 92–97 (1971).
47 Prange, A.J., Jr.; Wilson, I.C.; Lynn, C.W.; Alltop, L.B.; Stikeleather, R.A.: *L*-Tryptophan in mania. Archs. gen. Psychiat. *30:* 56–62 (1974).
48 Anath, J.: Treatment approaches to mania. Int. Pharmacopsychiat. *11:* 215–231 (1976).
49 Van Praag, H.M.; Korf, J.: 5-Hydroxytryptophan as an antidepressant. J. nerv. ment. Dis. *158:* 331–337 (1974).
50 Fugiwara, J.; Otsuki, S.: Subtype of affective psychosis classified by response on amine precursors and monoamine metabolism. Folia psychiat. neurol. Jap *28:* 93–99 (1974).
51 Van Praag, H.M.; Korf, J.: Für Diskussion: Central monoamine deficiency in depression: causative or secondary phenomenon? Pharmikopsychiatry *8:* 322–326 (1975).
52 Kline, N.S.; Sacks, W.: Relief of depression within one day using MAO inhibitor and intravenous 5-HTP. Am. J. Psychiat. *120:* 274–275 (1963).
53 Kline, N.S.; Sacks, W.; Simpson, G.M.: Further studies on: one day treatment of depression with 5-HPT. Am. J. Psychiat. *121:* 379–381 (1964).
54 Matussek, N.; Angst, J.; Benkert, O.; Gmur, M.; Papousek, M.; Ruther, E.; Waggon, B.: The effect of *L*-5-hydroxy-tryptophan alone and in combination with a decarboxylase inhibitor (RO4-4602) in depressive patients. Adv. Biochem. Psychopharmacol. *11:* 399–404 (1974).
55 Shaw, D.M.; Camps, F.E.; Eccleston, E.G.: 5-Hydroxy-tryptamine in the hindbrain of depressive suicides. Br. J. Psychiat. *113:* 1407–1411 (1967).
56 Bourne, H.R.; Bunney, W.E., Jr.; Colburn, R.W.; Davis, J.M.; David, J.M.; Shaw, D.M.; Coppen, A.J.: Noradrenaline, 5-hydroxytryptamine, and 5-hydroxyindoleacetic acid in hindbrains of suicidal patients. Lancet *ii:* 805–808 (1968).
57 Lloyd, K.G.; Farley, I.J.; Deck, J.H.N.; Horneykiewicz, O.: Serotonin and 5-hydroxyindoleacetic acid in discrete areas of the brain stems of suicidal victims and control patients. Adv. Biochem. Psychopharmacol. *11:* 387–397 (1974).
58 Asberg, M.; Traskman, L.; Thoren, P.: 5-HIAA in the cerebrospinal fluid: a biochemical suicide predictor? Archs. gen. Psychiat. *33:* 1193–1197 (1976).

59 Bunney, W.E.; Post, R.M.; Andersen, A.E.; Kopanda, R.T.: A neuronal receptor sensitivity mechanism in affective illness (a review of the evidence). Commun. Psychopharmacol. *1:* 393–405 (1977).
60 Fleisher, L.N.; Simon, J.R.; Aprison, M.H.: A biochemical-behavioral model for studying serotonergic supersensitivity in brain. J. Neurochem. *32:* 1613–1619 (1979).
61 Savage, D.D.; Mendels, J.; Frazer, A.: Monoamine oxidase inhibitors and serotonin uptake inhibitors: differential effects on [^{3}H]-serotonin binding sites in rat brain. J. Pharmac. exp. Ther. *212:* 259–263 (1979).
62 Wirz-Justice, A.; Krauchi, K.; Lichsteiner, M.; Feer, H.: Is it possible to modify serotonin receptor sensitivity? Life Sci. *23:* 1249–1254 (1978).
63 Sachar, E.J.; Finkelstein, J.; Hellman, L.: Growth hormone response in depressive illness. I. Response to insulin tolerance test. Archs. gen. Psychiat. *25:* 263–269 (1971).
64 Bivens, C.H.; Lebovitz, H.E.; Feldman, J.M.: Inhibition of hypoglycemia-induced growth hormone secretion by the serotonin antagonist cyproheptadine and methysergide. New Engl. J. Med. *289:* 236–239 (1973).
65 Brown, G.M.; Friend, W.C.; Chambers, J.W.: Neuropharmacology of hypothalamic-pituitary regulation; in Tolis, Clinical neuroendocrinology: a pathophysiologic approach, pp. 47–81 (Raven Press, New York 1979).
66 Prange, A.J.; Wilson, I.C.; Hara, P.P.; Alltop, L.B.; Breese, G.R.: Effects of thyrotropin-releasing hormone in depression. Lancet *ii:* 999–1002 (1972).
67 Kastin, A.J.; Ehrensing, R.H.; Schalch, D.S.; Andersen, M.S.: Improvement in mental depression with decreased thyrotropin response after administration of thyrotropin-releasing hormone. Lancet *ii:* 740–742 (1972).
68 Jordan, D.; Pigeon, P.; McRae-Degueurce, A.; Pujol, J.F.; Mornex, R.: Participation of serotonin in thyrotropin release. II. Evidence for the action of serotonin on the phasic release of thyrotropin. Endocrinology *105:* 975–979 (1979).
69 Carroll, B.J.; Curtis, G.S.; Mendels, J.: Neuroendocrine regulation in depression. I. Limbic system adrenocortical dysfunction. Archs. gen. Psychiat. *33:* 1039–1044 (1976).
70 Sachar, E.J.; Hellman, L.; Roffwarg, J.: Disrupted 24-hour patterns of cortisol secretion in psychotic depression. Archs. gen. Psychiat. *28:* 19–24 (1973).
71 Carroll, B.J.; Martin, F.I.R.; Davies, B.M.: Resistance to suppression by dexamethasone of plasma 11-hydroxycorticosteroid levels in severe depressive illness. Br. med. J. *iii:* 285–287 (1968).
72 Nuller, J.L.; Ostroumova, M.N.: Resistance to inhibiting effects of dexamethasone in patients with endogenous depression. Acta psychiat. scand. *61:* 169–177 (1980).
73 Scapagnini, U.; Moberg, G.P.; Van Loon, G.R.; De Groot, J.; Ganong, W.F.: Relation of brain 5-hydroxytryptamine content to diurnal variation in plasma corticosterone in the rat. Neuroendocrinology *7:* 90–96 (1971).
74 Mullen, P.E.; Silman, R.E.: The pineal and psychiatry: a review. Psychol. Med. *7:* 407–417 (1977).
75 Carman, J.S.; Post, R.M.; Buswell, R.; Goodwin, F.K.: Negative effects of melatonin on depression. Am. J. Psychiat. *133:* 1181–1186 (1976).

76 Kupfer, D.J.; Foster, F.G.; Coble, P.; McPartland, R.J.; Ulreck, R.F.: The application of EEG sleep for the differential diagnosis of affective disorders. Am. J. Psychiat. *135:* 69–74 (1978).

77 Wehr, T.A.; Wirz-Justice, A.; Goodwin, F.K.; Duncan, W.; Gillin, J.C.: Phase advance of the circadian sleep-wake cycle as an antidepressant. Science, N.Y. *206:* 710–713 (1979).

78 Wehr, T.A.; Goodwin, F.K.: Rapid cycling in manic-depressives induced by tricyclic antidepressants. Archs. gen. Psychiat. *36:* 555–559 (1979).

79 Johnson, A.; Pflug, B.; Engelmann, W.: Effect of lithium carbonate on circadian periodicity in humans. Pharmakopsychiatry *12:* 423–425 (1979).

Effects of Antidepressant Drugs on Adrenergic Responsiveness and Receptors

Alan Frazer and Joseph Mendels

The Fairmount Institute; Veterans Administration Hospital and Departments of Psychiatry and Pharmacology, University of Pennsylvania School of Medicine, Philadelphia, Pennsylvania

Different types of studies have demonstrated that antidepressant drugs exert prominent effects on monoamine-containing neurons in the brain. Thus, it has been postulated that affective illnesses are associated with some dysfunction of central monoamine-containing neuronal networks. The most prominent theories about the biology of major psychiatric diseases stem from observations on the effects of psychoactive drugs in animals rather than from studies showing biologic alterations in patients with mental diseases.

It is a fallacy to assume that information about the mechanism of action of a drug used to treat a disease *necessarily* provides insight into the etiology of the illness. However, given the limited accessibility to the patients' central nervous system, properly designed drug studies in animals may yield useful information and generate hypotheses about the underlying biology of mental illnesses. This chapter, then, will focus on the effects of antidepressants on monoamine-containing neurons in the brain, with particular attention to their effects on adrenergic responses.

Until recently, our understanding of how antidepressant drugs affect central monoamine-containing neuronal networks was based primarily on in vitro or on short-term in vivo experiments. Key observations revealed that tricyclic antidepressant drugs, such as imipramine, enhanced and prolonged responses elicited by monoamines, such as norepinephrine (NE) or 5-hydroxytryptamine (5HT; serotonin). Enhanced responsiveness was related to the ability of the tricyclic compounds to block the reuptake of NE or serotonin into nerve terminals [6, 9]. The uptake of these amines into the presynaptic nerve terminals from which they were released is the primary means of terminating their activity [17]. Based upon this and related pharmacologic observations, several theories of the genesis of affective disorders were formulated. Briefly, they considered depression to be associated with some functional deficiency present in monoamine-containing neurons in the brain [5, 7, 24, 27].

The theories described above failed to take into account the fact that antidepressants are given to patients for relatively long periods (weeks, months and occasionally years), often without loss of therapeutic effects. Indeed, there is a widely held clinical belief that a latent period of 7–20 days exists between the beginning of drug administration and the appearance of clinical improvement. Unfortunately, few studies can be marshalled to support this belief since many patients do not receive full dosages of the tricyclic drugs until at least several weeks after the initiation of therapy. Nevertheless, these clinical observations, coupled with the realization that monoamine neurons possess a variety of compensatory processes that can modify the initial effect of a drug, have caused a number of investigators to examine the effects of antidepressant drugs when given to animals, repeatedly, for a prolonged time. Frequently, the effects observed were different from those seen either in vitro or shortly after the administration of a single dose of the test drug.

Effect of Repeated Administration of Antidepressant Drugs on Adrenergic Responsiveness in Rats

Brain

Our group has been exploring this issue for several years. In particular, we have been examining whether repeated administration of antidepressant drugs affects noradrenergic responsiveness in the same way as acute treatment. We measured a response that is closely linked to the activation of adrenergic receptors.

From the elegant work of *Sutherland and Rall* [31] it was shown that an early response to activation of beta-adrenergic receptors by NE is the formation of adenosine 3'-,5'-monophosphate (cyclic AMP) by the enzyme adenylate cyclase (fig. 1). Cyclic AMP (formed in the cell) then initiates reactions which ultimately produce some type of cellular response, e.g., glycogenolysis, possibly membrane potential changes [3]. Catecholamines such as NE can stimulate cyclic AMP in brain tissue. Therefore, we measured the ability of NE to stimulate cyclic AMP in brain slices obtained from rats treated repeatedly with either imipramine, desmethylimipramine (DMI), or saline. Rather than the expected result (i.e., more cyclic AMP being formed in response to NE in tricyclic drug-treated rats), we found that the ability of NE to stimulate cyclic AMP was

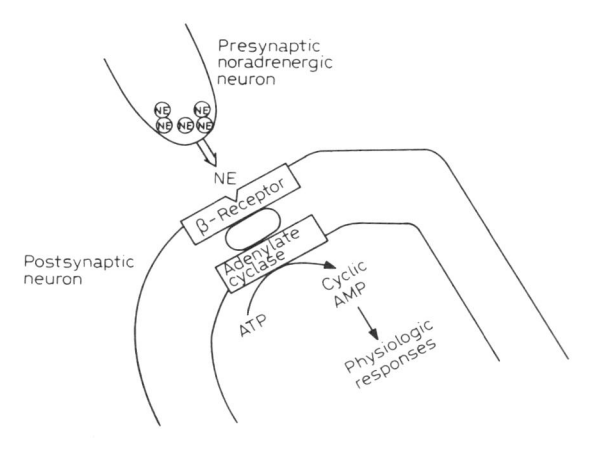

Fig. 1. Schematic representation of noradrenergic neuron stimulation of cyclic AMP in postsynaptic cell.

decreased in cerebral cortical slices prepared from chronically treated rats [10–12]. This decrease did not occur following a single injection of DMI.

Results similar to these have been obtained by *Vetulani and Sulser* [35] and *Vetulani* et al. [36, 37]. They showed that the inhibitory effect of chronic tricyclic treatment on noradrenergic responsiveness in limbic forebrain slices was mimicked by chronic administration of monoamine oxidase inhibitors, by the tricyclic-like antidepressant iprindole, and by electroconvulsive shocks. As with DMI treatment, acute administration of monoamine oxidase inhibitors, iprindole, or electroconvulsive shock produced no significant effect.

The positive result obtained with iprindole in this system deserves emphasis. This tricyclic-like antidepressant has little or no effect on either NE and serotonin uptake or metabolism, nor on monoamine oxidase activity [13, 25]. This led some investigators to question whether the standard tricyclic drugs exert their antidepressant activity by inhibiting monoamine uptake, or whether biogenic amines are at all involved in depression. Such speculation seems premature. Why should drugs modify the responses elicited by monoamine neurotransmitters only by either blocking their reuptake or inhibiting monoamine oxidase? It seems much more likely that multiple mechanisms can accomplish this. The demonstration by *Vetulani and Sulser* [35] and *Vetulani* et al. [36, 37] that iprindole possesses the ability to reduce noradrenergic responsiveness, like other antidepressants, substantiates such a view.

Pineal Gland

The reduced biochemical responsiveness to NE following chronic antidepressant treatment was shown only in in vitro studies. Therefore, it was important to determine whether such treatment also reduced or abolished noradrenergic responsiveness in vivo, especially in a system when acute treatment with a tricyclic drug produces enhancement of the NE effect.

The pineal gland of the rat is an excellent model system for testing these ideas. First, the pineal gland has a high density of beta-adrenergic receptors coupled to adenylate cyclase. Adenylate cyclase activation leads to increased concentrations of cyclic AMP in the gland [14, 39]. Second, the pineal gland lies outside the blood-brain barrier. As a consequence, it can respond to catecholamines added into the circulation. For these reasons, we treated rats, either acutely or repeatedly, with DMI and measured the ability of either NE or isoproterenol (administered intraperitoneally) to increase cyclic AMP levels in pineal glands [21]. The most salient features of this experiment are shown in figure 2. Intraperitoneal administration of NE did not increase pineal gland levels of cyclic AMP in control rats. However, NE caused a marked elevation of this nucleotide in rats given a single injection of DMI. Neither NE nor isoproterenol raised cyclic AMP concentrations in the pineal gland of rats treated repeatedly with DMI. Similarly, we recently found that isoproterenol is less effective in stimulating pineal cyclic AMP in rats treated for 5 consecutive days with the monoamine oxidase inhibitor nialamide [*Moyer* et al., in preparation].

The study described above highlights the difference between acute and repeated administration of antidepressant agents on noradrenergic responsiveness. Acute treatment with DMI potentiated the response elicited by NE, whereas repeated DMI treatment abolished noradrenergic responsiveness.

The pineal gland also is a useful model for studying responses elicited by endogenously released NE. This is because it receives its sole innervation from postganglionic sympathetic fibers originating from the superior cervical ganglion [19]. The activity of these nerves is influenced by environmental lighting. Darkness increases the activity of the noradrenergic fibers going to the pineal gland [4, 32]. Thus, it is possible to produce changes in the activity of the sympathetic nerve input to the pineal gland by exposing rats normally kept in light to darkness. We have done this with rats given either a single injection of DMI or multiple injections of this drug over 5 days [15].

As shown in figure 3, the pineal content of cyclic AMP was much higher in rats given a single injection of DMI and exposed to darkness than in rats given DMI and decapitated in the light. By contrast, rats treated with DMI for

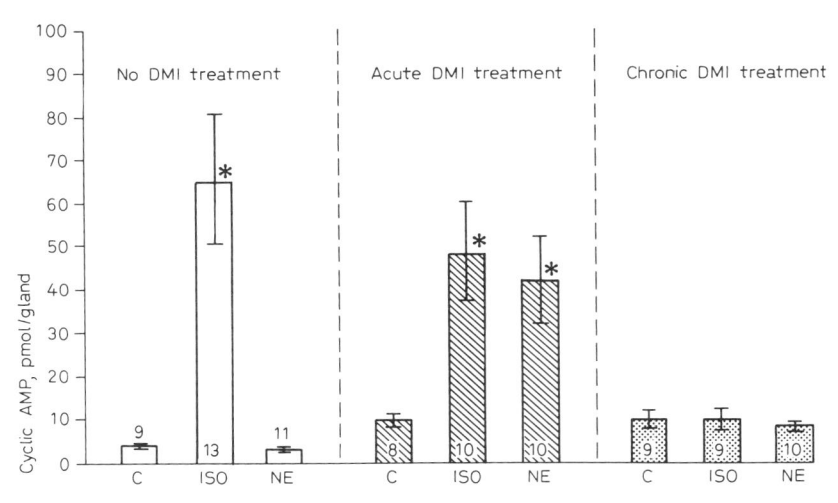

Fig. 2. Effect of DMI treatment on catecholamine-stimulated cyclic AMP production in the pineal gland in vivo. Two groups of rats were administered either saline or DMI (10 mg/kg, i.p.) twice daily for a total of 9 injections (5 days). A third group of rats (acute DMI treatment) received 8 injections of saline (days 1–4) followed by a single injection of DMI (10 mg/kg, i.p.) on day 5. 1 h after the final saline or DMI injection, rats were injected intraperitoneally with either 0.1% ascorbate (controls; C) or isoproterenol (ISO; 2 μmol/kg) and were decapitated 2.5 min later. Pineal glands were removed within 30 s of decapitation, sonicated in 1 ml of 2.5% perchloric acid, and assayed for cyclic AMP. Values represent the mean ± SEM of the number of rats indicated. Asterisks indicate values significantly different from those measured in corresponding control rats (student's t test, two-tailed, $p < 0.025$). (NE = additional control group injected with norepinephrine.)
(Reprinted by permission from J.A. Moyer et al.: "Opposite effects of acute and repeated administration of desmethylimipramine on adrenergic responsiveness in rat pineal gland," *Life Sciences*, Vol. 24, pp. 2237–2244. Copyright 1979, Pergamon Press, Ltd., New York.)

5 days showed no rise in pineal cyclic AMP upon exposure to darkness (fig. 3). In a separate study [16], we demonstrated that the rise in pineal cyclic AMP caused by exposure to darkness in DMI-treated rats results from NE activation of pineal beta-adrenergic receptors, with NE being released from the sympathetic nerve innervating the gland.

Thus, regardless of the way in which noradrenergic responsiveness is elicited, either by in vitro addition of NE to brain slices, by exogenous administration of catecholamines in vivo, or by darkness-induced alterations in the release of NE from sympathetic nerve terminals, treatment of rats with DMI causes a reduction in beta-adrenergic responsiveness.

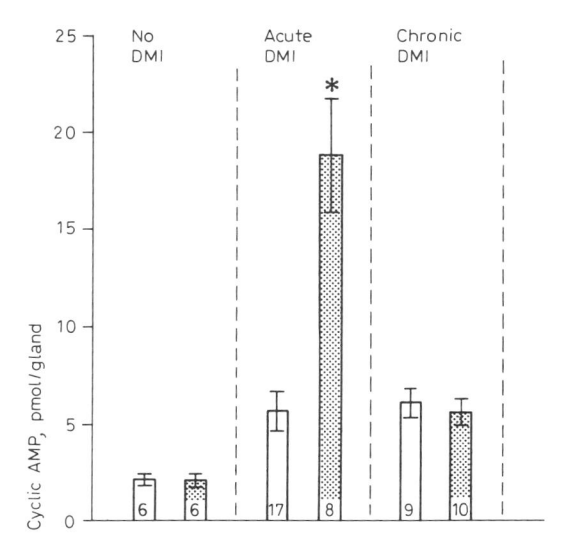

Fig. 3. Effect of acute and repeated administration of DMI on pineal gland cyclic AMP in rats exposed to the dark. Rats received either a single injection of DMI (10 mg/kg) or 9 injections of the drug over 5 days. 1 h after the final saline or DMI injection, the rats were either kept in the light (open bars) or exposed to darkness (dotted bars) for 1 min. Each bar and bracket represent the mean value ± SEM, respectively. The figures in each bar show the number of experiments. Only rats that received a single injection of DMI before exposure to darkness had higher values of pineal cyclic AMP than that measured in corresponding rats kept in the light ($p < 0.001$).

Adrenergic Receptor Binding Sites after Repeated Administration of Antidepressants

What is the mechanism for the diminution in noradrenergic responsiveness seen after repeated administration of drugs like DMI? The development of techniques that measure the binding of a drug to a receptor helps us answer this question. Before this development, it was possible only to infer some alteration in receptor properties by measuring the result of the drug interaction with the receptor, i.e., a response. Now, radioactive compounds that bind to physiologic receptors are available commercially. Many of these compounds satisfy criteria for binding to specific physiologic receptors. The use of radiolabeled compounds that bind to physiologic receptors has enabled investigators to probe the molecular events associated with changes in receptor properties [20].

Our interest in measuring adrenergic receptor binding sites, i.e., to explain why chronic antidepressant treatment reduces beta-adrenergic responsiveness, arose from the well-known observation that the amount of prior exposure of an organ to certain stimulants can exert a strong influence on the magnitude of the response elicited by subsequent administration of the stimulant. For example, denervation of skeletal muscle leads to an increased responsiveness to acetylcholine [1], i.e., supersensitivity to acetylcholine. With the use of receptor binding techniques [23] it was demonstrated that on skeletal muscle this increased responsiveness was associated with a rise in receptor binding sites for acetylcholine. Thus, little or no exposure of skeletal muscle to acetylcholine results in an increased responsiveness of the tissue to acetylcholine. This is due, at least in part, to a greater than normal number of acetylcholine receptors contained in the muscle. Similar results have been obtained upon denervation of organs receiving noradrenergic innervation [30, 34, 38]. Drug-induced increases in receptor number may be responsible for certain drug effects, e.g., tardive dyskinesia caused by administration of neuroleptics [29].

In contrast to the increased responsiveness observed after denervation, prolonged exposure of an organ to a stimulant results in diminished responsiveness. Following subsequent exposure to the stimulant, there will be a decreased organ response. This phenomenon is called subsensitivity and has been observed in cholinergic [33] and adrenergic systems [8, 18]. This decline in responsiveness has been shown to be associated with a reduction in receptor binding sites [22, 23].

In summary, organs (including brain) modify their responsiveness to cholinergic or adrenergic stimulation in a manner inversely related to their prior exposure to acetylcholine or NE. Little prior exposure leads to increased responsiveness, whereas overexposure causes decreased responsiveness. The alteration in sensitivity occurs because of a change in the density of receptor sites. This is shown schematically in figure 4.

With this in mind, it seemed possible that chronic antidepressant drug treatment increased the exposure of beta-adrenergic receptors to NE as a consequence of either blockade of the reuptake of NE or monoamine oxidase inhibition. The increased exposure of the receptors to NE, in turn, causes a decrease in beta-adrenergic receptor density. This produces the decreased responsiveness measured after repeated antidepressant treatment. A number of investigators, who reported decreased numbers of beta-adrenergic binding sites in rat brain [2, 26, 40] and pineal gland [21] following antidepressant drug treatment, have substantiated this idea.

As shown in table I, many different types of antidepressant treatments, when given repeatedly to rats, lower beta-adrenergic receptor binding sites in the brain. Some treatments, like iprindole or electroconvulsive shocks, have

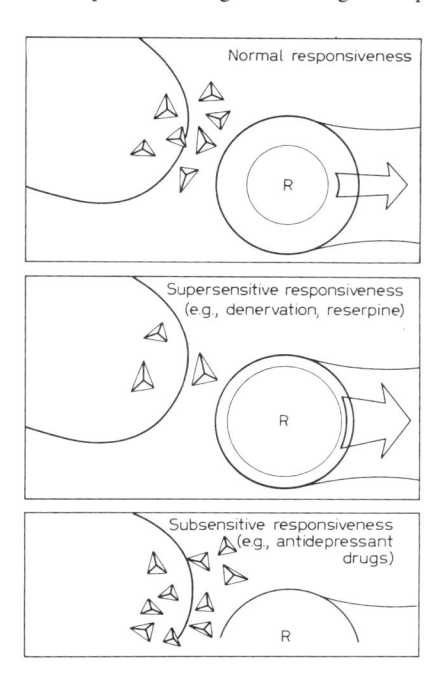

Fig. 4. Changes in beta-adrenergic responsiveness mediated through alterations in beta-adrenergic receptor density.

Table 1. Effect of antidepressant treatments on NE uptake, monoamine oxidase activity, or beta-adrenergic receptors

Antidepressant treatment	Effect on NE uptake	Monoamine oxidase	Beta-adrenergic binding sites
Tricyclics			
Amitriptyline	+	0	+
Chlorimipramine	+	0	+
DMI	+	0	+
Doxepin	+	0	+
Nortriptyline	+	0	+
Iprindole	0	0	+
Monoamine oxidase inhibitors			
Nialamide	0	+	+
Pargyline	0	+	+
Tranylcypromine	0	+	+
Electroconvulsive therapy	0	0	+

this action even when they have little or no effect on NE uptake or on monoamine oxidase. Furthermore, it has been shown [28] that treatment of rats with psychoactive drugs that do not ameliorate the core symptomatology of depression (e.g., L-dopa, diazepam, antihistamines, major tranquilizers, or cocaine) do not cause any significant reduction in beta-adrenergic binding sites in the brain. Thus, many antidepressant treatments produce a decrease in beta-adrenergic receptor sites in the brain over time. This effect is caused selectively by antidepressant drugs and electroconvulsive therapy and is not present with nonantidepressant drugs.

A key question relates to whether the increase in beta-adrenergic receptors, with a concomitant reduction in adrenergic responsiveness, is related to the antidepressant properties of these treatments. Unfortunately, this question can currently not be answered, since clinical studies exploring this phenomenon have yet to be initiated. Nevertheless, these data highlight the complex, multiple effects produced by antidepressant treatments at the adrenergic synapse. Accordingly, we believe that current theories which hold that antidepressants exert their clinical effects by acutely enhancing noradrenergic responses should be reevaluated, and consideration should be given to the possibility that some of their therapeutic actions may, in fact, be due to a decrease in adrenergic reactivity.

References

1 Axelsson, J.; Thesleff, S.: A study of supersensitivity in denervated mammalian skeletal muscle. J. Physiol., Lond. *147:* 178–193 (1959).
2 Banerjee, S.P.; Kung, L.S.; Riggi, S.J.; et al.: Development of β-adrenergic receptor subsensitivity by antidepressants. Nature, Lond. *268:* 455–456 (1977).
3 Bloom, F.E.: Cyclic nucleotides in central synaptic function. Fed. Proc. *38:* 2203–2207 (1979).
4 Brownstein, M.; Axelrod, J.: Pineal gland: 24-hour rhythm in norepinephrine turnover. Science *184:* 163–165 (1974).
5 Bunney, W.E., Jr.; Davis, J.M.: Norepinephrine in depressive reactions. A review. Archs. gen. Psychiat. *13:* 483–494 (1965).
6 Carlsson, A.; Fuxe, K.; Ungerstedt, U.: The effect of imipramine on central 5-hydroxytryptamine neurons. J. Pharm. Pharmac. *20:* 150–151 (1968).
7 Coppen, A.: The biochemistry of affective disorders. Br. J. Psychiat. *113:* 1237–1264 (1967).
8 Deguchi, T.; Axelrod, J.: Supersensitivity and subsensitivity of the β-adrenergic receptor in pineal gland regulated by catecholamine transmitter. Proc. natn. Acad. Sci. USA *70:* 2411–2414 (1973).
9 Dengler, H.J.; Speigel, H.E.; Titus, E.O.: Effects of drugs on uptake of isotopic norepinephrine by cat tissues. Nature, Lond. *191:* 816–817 (1961).

10 Frazer, A.; Mendels, J.: Do tricyclic antidepressants enhance adrenergic transmission? Am. J. Psychiat. *134:* 1040–1042 (1977).
11 Frazer, A.; Hess, M.E.; Mendels, J.; et al.: Influence of acute and chronic treatment with desmethylimipramine on catecholamine effects in the rat. J. Pharmac. exp. Ther. *206:* 311–319 (1978).
12 Frazer, A.; Pandey, G.; Mendels, J.; et al.: The effect of tri-iodothyronine on [^{3}H]-cyclic AMP production in slices of rat cerebral cortex. Neuropharmacology *13:* 1131–1140 (1974).
13 Gluckman, M.I.; Baum, T.: The pharmacology of iprindole, a new antidepressant. Psychopharmacologia, Berlin *15:* 169–185 (1969).
14 Greenberg, L.H.; Weiss, B.: β-Adrenergic receptors in aged rat brain: reduced number and capacity of pineal gland to develop supersensitivity. Science *201:* 61–63 (1978).
15 Heydorn, W.; Mendels, J.; Frazer, A.: Do tricyclic antidepressants enhance adrenergic transmission? An update. Am. J. Psychiat. *137:* 113–114 (1980).
16 Heydorn, W.E.; Mendels, J.; Frazer, A.: Effect of darkness and of desmethylimipramine on pineal gland concentrations of cyclic AMP. Biochem. Pharmac. (in press).
17 Iversen, L.: Role of transmitter uptake mechanism in synaptic neurotransmission. Br. J. Pharmacol. *41:* 571–591 (1971).
18 Kakiuchi, S.; Rall, T.W.: The influence of chemical agents on the accumulation of adenosine 3′,5′-phosphate in slices of rabbit cerebellum. Molec. Pharmacol. *4:* 367–378 (1968).
19 Kappers, J.A.: The development, topographical relations and innervation of the epiphysis cerebri in the albino rat. Z. Zellforsch. mikrosk. Anat. *52:* 163–215 (1960).
20 Lefkowitz, R.J.; Williams, L.T.: Molecular mechanisms of activation and desensitization of adenylate cyclase coupled beta-adrenergic receptors. Adv. cyclic Nucleotide Res. *9:* 1–17 (1978).
21 Moyer, J.A.; Greenberg, L.H.; Frazer, A.; et al.: Opposite effects of acute and repeated administration of desmethylimipramine on adrenergic responsiveness in rat pineal gland. Life Sci. *24:* 2237–2244 (1979).
22 Mukherjee, C.; Caron, M.G.; Lefkowitz, R.J.: Catecholamine-induced subsensitivity of adenylate cyclase associated with loss of β-adrenergic receptor binding sites. Proc. natn. Acad. Sci. USA *72:* 1946–1949 (1975).
23 Potter, L.; Miledi, R.: Acetylcholine receptors in muscle fibers. Nature, Lond. *233:* 599–603 (1971).
24 Prange, A.J., Jr.: The pharmacology and biochemistry of depression. Dis. nerv. Syst. *25:* 217–221 (1964).
25 Ross, S.B.; Renyi, A.L.; Ogren, S.O.: A comparison of the inhibitory activities of iprindole and imipramine on the uptake of 5-hydroxytryptamine and noradrenaline in brain slices. Life Sci. *10:* 1267–1277 (1971).
26 Sarai, K.; Frazer, A.; Brunswick, D.; et al.: Desmethyl-imipramine-induced decrease in β-adrenergic receptor binding in rat cerebral cortex. Biochem. Pharmac. *27:* 2179–2181 (1978).
27 Schildkraut, J.J.: The catecholamine hypothesis of affective disorders: a review of supporting evidence. Am. J. Psychiat. *122:* 509–522 (1965).

28 Sellinger-Barnette, M.M.; Mendels, J.; Frazer, A.: The effect of psychoactive drugs on beta-adrenergic receptor binding sites in rat brain. Neuropharmacology (in press).

29 Snyder, S.H.: Receptors, neurotransmitters and drug responses. New Engl. J. Med. *300:* 465–472 (1979).

30 Sporn, J.R.; Harden, T.K.; Wolfe, B.B.; et al.: β-Adrenergic receptor involvement in 6-hydroxydopamine-induced supersensitivity in rat cerebral cortex. Science *194:* 624–626 (1976).

31 Sutherland, E.W.; Rall, T.W.: The relation of adenosine-3',5'-phosphate and phosphorylase to the actions of catecholamines and other hormones. Pharmac. Rev. *12:* 265–299 (1960).

32 Taylor, A.; Wilson, R.: Electrophysiological evidence for the action of light on the pineal gland in the rat. Experientia *26:* 267–269 (1970).

33 Thesleff, S.: The mode of action of neuromuscular block caused by acetylcholine, nicotine, decamethonium, and succinylcholine. Acta physiol. scand. *34:* 218–231 (1955).

34 Trendelenburg, U.: Mechanism of supersensitivity and subsensitivity to sympathomimetic amines. Pharmac. Rev. *18:* 629–640 (1966).

35 Vetulani, J.; Sulser, F.: Action of various antidepressant treatments reduces reactivity of noradrenergic cyclic AMP-generating system in limbic forebrain. Nature, Lond. *257:* 495–496 (1975).

36 Vetulani, J.; Stawarz, R.J.; Dingell, J.V.; et al.: A possible common mechanism of action of antidepressant treatments. Arch. Pharmacol. *293:* 109–114 (1976).

37 Vetulani, J.; Stawarz, R.J.; Sulser, F.: Adaptative mechanisms of the noradrenergic cyclic AMP generating system in the limbic forebrain of the rat: adaptation to persistent changes in the availability of norepinephrine (NE). J. Neurochem. *27:* 661–666 (1976).

38 Weiss, B.; Costa, E.: Adenyl cyclase activity in rat pineal gland: effects of chronic denervation and norepinephrine. Science *156:* 1750–1752 (1967).

39 Weiss, B.; Costa, E.: Selective stimulation of adenyl cyclase of rat pineal gland by pharmacologically active catecholamines. J. Pharmac. exp. Ther. *161:* 310–319 (1968).

40 Wolfe, B.B.; Harden, T.K.; Sporn, J.R.; et al.: Presynaptic modulation of beta-adrenergic receptors in rat cerebral cortex after treatment with antidepressants. J. Pharmac. exp. Ther. *207:* 446–457 (1978).

The Psychobiology of Affective Disorders. Pfizer Symp. Depression, Boca Raton 1980, pp. 83–98 (Karger, Basel 1980)

The Cholinergic Nervous System and Depression

David S. Janowsky*

Mental Health Clinical Research Center, Veterans Administration Medical Center; Department of Psychiatry, University of California, San Diego, California

It has been hypothesized that affective disorders are determined by a complex balance between cholinergic and adrenergic neurotransmitters, with a relative imbalance between central adrenergic and cholinergic neurotransmitter activity existing in those areas of the brain that regulate affect. Thus, depression has been postulated to be a disease of central cholinergic predominance, relative to norepinephrine and/or dopamine, and mania has been postulated as the converse [1]. At the time that the cholinergic-adrenergic hypothesis of affective disorders was proposed, study of the role of cholinergic factors in emotional disorders was a relatively neglected area of investigation. The most popular neurotransmitter hypotheses focused extensively on the role of norepinephrine, serotonin, or, to a lesser extent, dopamine as the regulatory chemicals of mania and depression. The following is a review of the pertinent literature which indicates that acetylcholine, like serotonin, dopamine and norepinephrine, may be important in the regulation of affect.

The philosophic basis for the cholinergic-adrenergic hypothesis of affective disorders derives from the concept that neurotransmitters rarely act alone with respect to endocrine and autonomic function. Perhaps the most classic example of a balance between neurotransmitter systems is found in the autonomic nervous system, in which peripherally and/or centrally mediated adrenergic-cholinergic balance regulates such diverse functions as heart rate, gastrointestinal motility, pupillary size, and blood pressure. Based on this knowledge, it was reasoned that like a variety of peripheral autonomic functions and like the central regulation of extrapyramidal symptoms, mood may be regulated by a balance or interaction between catecholaminergic and cholinergic factors, rather

*In association with Craig Risch, Leighton Huey, Donald Parker, John Davis and Lewis Judd than that depression and mania represent, respectively, too little or too much of a given neurotransmitter. Because of this conceptualization, investigators have been able to apply a variety of concepts relevant to autonomic regulation and disregulation to the study of affective disorders.

Animal Behavioral Studies

As reviewed elsewhere [1], a number of animal studies have been supportive of the cholinergic-adrenergic hypothesis of affective disorders. To mention a few, increasing central cholinergic activity by a variety of cholinomimetic drugs causes behavioral depressant-inhibitory effects on such animal measures of antidepressant activity as locomotion and self-stimulation, and causes antagonism of methylphenidate-induced stereotype behavior [2]. Anticholinergic agents cause the opposite effects [1]. Also, the antiadrenergic drug reserpine causes effects in animals that parallel those of cholinomimetic agonists. Like cholinomimetic agents, reserpine causes peripheral parasympathetic effects as well as decreased locomotor activity, decreased self-stimulation, decreased conditioned responses, and antagonism and methylphenidate-induced, stereotype gnawing behavior [1, 3].

Cholinergic-Anticholinergic Effects of Depressants and Antidepressants

In man, all antiadrenergic agents, including propranolol, alphamethyldopa, and reserpine, have parasympathetic side effects [4]. Furthermore, the psychologic side effects of reserpine are remarkably similar to those occurring after exposure to centrally acting cholinomimetic agents (i.e. depression, nightmares, lethargy, anergy, sleepiness). Thus, the behavioral effects of reserpine and other antiadrenergic agents could be explained on the basis of their central cholinomimetic as well as their antiadrenergic effects [1, 3]. Conversely, most effective antidepressant treatments suppress acetylcholine activity, either by exerting antimuscarinic effects or by decreasing acetylcholine turnover. Although the tricyclic antidepressants' ability to elevate mood in depressed patients and occasionally to induce mania has been attributed to their ability to increase monoamine availability, imipramine and amitriptyline also have prominent central anticholinergic effects, causing a reversible, toxic, confusional state similar to that seen with atropine or scopolamine poisoning. Thus, tricyclic antidepressants block central cholinergic activity as well as shift the cholinergic-adrenergic balance toward an adrenergic predominance [1]. Unfortunately, however, anticholinergic agents such as atropine and scopolamine are not particularly effective antidepressants and there does not seem to be an obvious relationship between the degree of central anticholinergic activity of a given tricyclic antidepressant and its clinical efficacy or potency [3].

Effects of Cholinomimetic Agents in Man

The most convincing evidence that central cholinergic activity plays a significant role in the regulation of affect comes from studies of the psychologic effects of cholinesterase inhibitors in man. By inhibiting acetylcholinesterase, these agents inhibit the breakdown of acetylcholine and, thus, cause its buildup in the brain.

In 1950, *Rowntree* et al. [5] administered the irreversible cholinesterase inhibitor, diisopropylfluorophosphonate (DFP) to normal subjects and to manic depressive patients. Normal subjects developed lassitude, irritability, apathy, depression, and slowness or poverty of thoughts which appeared before the onset of peripheral cholinergic symptoms. Two remitted manic depressive patients showed mental changes similar to the normal subjects, while 2 hypomanic patients improved with DFP. Another hypomanic patient showed decreased manic symptoms and was minimally depressed after each of two courses of DFP. This patient relapsed upon DFP withdrawal. One almost remitted hypomanic patient became floridly manic upon DFP withdrawal. Also, 1 depressed patient showed a significant increase in depression during DFP administration. In 1961, *Gershon and Shaw* [6] reported on individuals poisoned with cholinesterase-inhibitor insecticides. Among other symptoms, these patients developed depression as well as peripheral parasympathetic toxicity. *Gershon and Shaw* [6] also noted a higher incidence of depression in those orchardists exposed to cholinesterase-inhibitor insecticides. Still later, *Bowers* et al. [7] noted that the irreversible cholinesterase inhibitor EA01701 caused depressed mood, decreased energy and enthusiasm, lethargy, and decreased friendliness in normal volunteers to whom it was given.

Similar to the above, studies with cholinesterase inhibitors in the early 1970s, intravenous physosigtmine (a reversible cholinesterase inhibitor which is centrally acting) and neostigmine (a similar cholinesterase inhibitor which does not cross the blood-brain barrier) were used by *Janowsky* et al. [1, 8] to study central cholinergic mechanisms in affect-disorder patients.

General Central Cholinergic Effects

In several studies, physostigmine was found to rapidly exert brief (1–2 h) behavioral effects in virtually all subjects who received it, consisting of many aspects of the psychomotor retardation component of depression, including lethargy, anergy, feelings of tiredness, motor retardation, feelings of being drained, and social withdrawal. This physostigmine inhibitory state usually preceded sensations of nausea or episodes of vomiting, and the entire syndrome could be antagonized by centrally acting anticholinergic agents, such as atropine or scopolamine [1, 3, 8].

Effects of Physostigmine on Manic Symptoms

In addition to its general inhibitory effects, physostigmine exerted significant antimanic effects in hypomanic and manic patients [1, 3], who, at baseline, exhibited typical manic symptoms, such as rapidity of thought and speech, grandiose ideation, euphoria, and rhyming. Administration of physostigmine to these patients, in most cases, resulted in a dramatic reduction of manic symptoms, whereas placebo and neostigmine produced no such changes. Thus, physostigmine rapidly converted the manic syndrome to a state consistent with a psychomotor-retarded depression. Patients appeared lethargic as well as slowed in their movements. They were significantly less talkative, euphoric, active, cheerful, happy, friendly, or grandiose, and had a decrease in flight of ideas. Patients also reported general inhibitory symptoms, such as feeling drained, being without energy, becoming apathetic, and having no thoughts. Often, the manic patients' responses included depression, with crying, sadness, and similar signs of depressed affect.

The observation that physostigmine decreases manic symptoms was confirmed subsequently by others. Two of 4 manic patients studied by *Modestin* et al. [9, 10] showed a lessening of manic symptoms following physostigmine administration, and a patient of *Carroll* et al. [11] showed psychomotor retardation. More recently, *Davis* et al. [12] reported that physostigmine had significant and dramatic antimanic effects in those manic patients who showed low, as opposed to high, anger and irritability levels.

In addition to antagonizing manic symptoms, a subsequent rebound into hypermania has been observed in some manic patients given physostigmine. *Shopsin* et al. [13] studied physostigmine's effects on 3 severely manic patients given relatively high intravenous doses of physostigmine. Although all 3 patients initially became somewhat anergic after receiving physostigmine, in 2 subjects a rebound into a "hypermanic state" occurred approximately 2 h following physostigmine administration which lasted up to 4 h and consisted of a marked exacerbation and intensification beyond the baseline levels of the mania. This was postulated to be an adrenergic compensation for the cholinergic overactivity.

Effects of Physostigmine on Depressive Symptoms

In addition to its nonspecific inhibitory-anergic and antimanic effects, physostigmine, but not neostigmine, is capable of inducing a depressed mood, consisting of such symptoms as sadness, feelings of uselessness, and intensification of suicidal feelings [3, 8]. Thus, depressed mood, as contrasted with more pervasive, nonspecific anergic-inhibitory effects, can occur following physostigmine infusion, and this effect seems to occur predominantly in manic or depressed manic depressive and unipolar depressed patients. In confirmation of these observations, *Davis* et al. [12] noted the frequent occurrence of depressed mood in manic patients following physostigmine infusion; and *Modestin* et al. [9, 10], in their sample of depressed patients, manic patients, and nonpsychotic, nondepressed control patients, noted that physostigmine produced a statistically significant overall increase in depressive symptomatology.

Data from *Modestin* et al. [9, 10] also are helpful in clarifying whether the depressive symptoms noted following physostigmine infusion are secondary to physostigmine's physical side effects, such as nausea and vomiting. If physostigmine-induced depressive symptoms are a consequence of physical symptoms, one would expect a correlation between the intensity of depressive symptoms and physical symptoms. When the results of *Modestin* et al. [9, 10] are summarized, there is no such correlation. Also, it has been observed that physostigmine's anergic-depressant effects precede, rather than follow or occur simultaneously with, its emetic and nausea-inducing effects. Thus, it is likely that physostigmine-induced depression is not caused simply by feeling physically ill [1, 3].

Marijuana-Physostigmine Interactions

In addition to causing a mild and short-lived depressive syndrome, *El-Yousef* et al. [14] noted that prior intoxication with marijuana intensified physostigmine's mood-depressing effects in normal subjects. Two marijuana-intoxicated normal volunteers who received physostigmine rapidly ceased to feel high and became profoundly depressed, expressing an extremely depressed mood, massive psychomotor retardation, and suicidal ideation. This dramatic induction of depression was reversed by atropine. Parallel subsequent animal-toxicity experiments have shown that Δ9-tetrahydrocannabinol enhances physostigmine's lethality in rodents [15]. The finding that a combination of marijuana and physostigmine may cause significant depression was replicated naturalistically by *Davis* et al. [16]. In contrast to other normal subjects, one who received physostigmine in a study of the cognitive effects of acetylcholine became quite depressed. It was learned later that this subject had smoked marijuana prior to the experiment.

Depressant Effects of Acetylcholine Precursors

Consistent with the mood-depressant effects of physostigmine in patients with an affective component to their illness, and of physostigmine plus marijuana in normal subjects, several anecdotal reports suggest that the presumed acetylcholine precursors deanol and choline may, in some cases, cause a depressed mood. *Tamminga* et al. [17] reported that choline administration caused an atropine-reversible, severe, depressed mood in 2 of 4 tardive dyskinesia patients to whom it was given. *Davis* [18] also noted that choline-treated schizophrenics report significantly more depressive symptoms than when treated with placebo. *Casey* [19] observed depressed mood in some and hypomania in others as a side effect in tardive dyskinesia patients who developed affective symptoms after a high dosage of deanol was administered.

Depression-Related Effects of Cholinomimetics

Some indirect observations further link the cholinergic nervous system with depression. *Sitarm* et al. [20] have observed that one of the major sleep defects in depression (shortened rapid eye movement, or REM, latency) resembles that caused by cholinomimetic drugs. *Kupfer* et al. [27] have shown that early reversal of this cholinergically mediated sleep variable in depressives predicts tricyclic antidepressant responsiveness. In addition, *Carroll* et al. [22] have shown that the ability of dexamethasone to suppress cortisol levels is antagonized by physostigmine, a finding that parallels the specific inability of dexamethasone to suppress cortisol secretion in patients with endogenous depression.

Differential Sensitivity of Affect-Disorder Patients to Cholinomimetic Drugs

There is a growing body of evidence that affect-disorder patients may be differentially more vulnerable to the effects of cholinomimetics than are nonaffect-disorder patients. If such phenomena were true, this would be specifically supportive of a role for cholinergic mechanisms in affect disorders and might be of clinical diagnostic usefulness. In a limited pilot study in 1973, *Janowsky,* et al. [3, 8] noted that while most patients became anergic after receiving physostigmine, depressives, manics, and schizoaffectives, in contrast to schizophrenics, became sadder, more tearful, and depressed. Furthermore, *Davis* et al. [16] noted that normal subjects receiving physostigmine became nauseated and anergic but did not become depressed. *Oppenheimer* et al. [23] observed that a significant proportion of euthymic manic depressive patients receiving lithium became depressed after receiving physostigmine, in contrast to drug-free normal subjects who also received physostigmine. Similarly, *Casey* [19] observed that only patients with a strong history of affective disorder showed affective symptoms while receiving deanol for tardive dyskinesia. More recently, *Sitarm* et al. [20] found that REM latency, an acetylcholine-sensitive sleep variable, decreased more in affect-disorder patients than in normal subjects following infusion of the cholinergic agent, arecholine. He has noted that this supersensitivity to a cholinomimetic drug occurs regardless of whether the patient has remitted clinically, or whether the patient has been drug-free for a period of months.

In 1980, *Janowsky* et al. [24] began more systematically to explore the possibility that physostigmine has differential behavioral effects in affect- and nonaffect-disorder patients. They have made significant progress in defining the differential behavioral effects of low dosage physostigmine in various patient groups. The 37 patients studied to date were adult men and nonpregnant women who were Veterans Administration Hospital psychiatric inpatients. They were in good health and between 18 and 55 years of age. Each subject was given a Schedule of Affect Disorder and Schizophrenia interview and the subsequent assignment of Research Diagnostic Criteria as well as a DSM-III diagnosis.

Patients were divided into 2 groups consisting of 11 affective disorder patients (7 with major depressive disorder and 4 with bipolar depression with mania) and 28 patients with other diagnoses (4 patients with schizoaffective disorder; 10 patients with alcoholism who had been detoxified; 2 who had a drug-use disorder; 2 with another psychiatric disorder diagnosis).

All were kept medication-free for at least 1 week. After having been kept without food or water for at least 8 h, at approximately 9 A.M., each test subject received an intramuscular injection of 1.0 mg methscopolamine to protect against the peripheral side effects of physostigmine (methscopolamine does not cross the blood-brain barrier). Twenty min later, each subject received, over a 10-min period, on a double-blind basis and in counterbalanced order, 0.022 mg/kg intravenous physostigmine salicylate on 1 day and matched placebo 1–4 days before or after. A crossover design was used with the patient as his own control.

Behavioral variables used to evaluate mood and inhibition in the study were: (1) The Hamilton Depression Rating Scale; (2) The Janowsky-Davis Activation-Inhibition (A-I) Scale [3]; (3) The Beigel-Murphy Mania Rating Scale; (4) The Brief Psychiatric Rating Scale; (5) The Profile of Mood States, and (6) The Beck Depression Rating Scale. These were administered 15 min before the start of physostigmine infusion and 10, 30, 45 and 60 min after completion of the infusion.

Data were collated and items and scales analyzed by means of analysis of variance techniques for within-subject and between-subject differences, using drug and diagnosis as variables.

The results of this study are outlined in tables I and II. Overall, physostigmine caused a number of statistically significant effects. Decreases were observed on the Beigel-Murphy Arousal-Activation subscale, the Euphoria-Grandiosity subscale, and the Beigel-Murphy Total Mania Scale as were significant increases on the NIMH Anergia and Depression subscales and the NIMH Total Scale score. On the A-I Scale, rater-evaluated and self-rated inhibition and dysphoria increased; activation decreased. Self-rated POMS Vigor and Elation and Friendliness subscales significantly decreased, and Tension-Anxiety, Depression-Dejection, Anger-Hostility, Fatigue and Confusion-Bewilderment subscales significantly increased.

Physostigmine effectively differentiated the affective-disorder patients and the other psychiatric patients on a number of variables. Generally, behavioral hyper-responsiveness was noted in the affective-disorder patients, compared with nonaffective-disorder patients. Thus, BPRS depression and total score ratings, rater-evaluated activation, inhibition, dysphoria, self-rated inhibition and POMS tension-anxiety, anger-hostility and fatigue, increased more, and friendliness decreased more in the affect-disorder patients.

Table 1. Behavioral and neuroendocrine effects of physostigmine compared with placebo in a group of psychiatric patients [1]

	Preinfusion	10 min. postinfusion
Rater Beigel-Murphy Mania Rating Scale		
Arousal	5.9 ± 0.5	4.5 ± 0.5†
Euphoria-grandiosity	2.8 ± 0.4	0.9 ± 0.3‡
Irritation	1.7 ± 0.4	2.7 ± 0.5*
Total	10.4 ± 1.0	7.7 ± 1.0†
Rater BPRS (NIMH)		
Anergia	5.6 ± 0.3	9.1 ± 0.6‡
Depression	6.6 ± 0.3	10.3 ± 0.5‡
Total	33.9 ± 1.2	43.3 ± 0.16‡
Rater Activation-Inhibition		
Inhibition	5.6 ± 1.1	23.9 ± 2.7‡
Activation	9.3 ± 0.4	5.3 ± 0.6‡
Dysphoria	1.3 ± 0.3	3.8 ± 0.5‡
Subject Activation-Inhibition		
Inhibition	15.8 ± 3.1	31.0 ± 3.5‡
Activation	10.3 ± 0.9	7.4 ± 1.0†
Dysphoria	2.4 ± 0.6	4.9 ± 0.9†
Subject POMS		
Tension-anxiety	9.7 ± 1.4	16.5 ± 2.1‡
Depression-dejection	15.7 ± 3.1	20.8 ± 3.6*
Anger-hostility	8.0 ± 2.4	11.1 ± 2.4*
Fatigue	4.7 ± 1.2	11.5 ± 1.6‡
Confusion-bewilderment	7.9 ± 1.3	12.9 ± 1.5‡
Vigor	12.8 ± 1.5	7.2 ± 1.3‡
Elation	8.2 ± 1.2	5.0 ± 1.1‡
Friendliness	17.0 ± 1.6	11.9 ± 1.6*
Neuroendocrines		
Growth hormone	0.94 ± 0.26	4.16 ± 1.63†
Cortisol	100 ± 6	217 ± 17‡
Prolactin	6.2 ± 0.4	25 ± 5.4‡

[1] All p values represent a comparison of the active physostigmine and placebo condition. *$p<0.05$; †$p<0.01$; ‡$p<0.001$.

Thus, physostigmine, again in a well-controlled study using rater and self-rated variables, has been shown to cause anergy as well as negative affect, including depressed mood. Furthermore, affective-disorder patients appear to be relatively more vulnerable to the cholinergic effects of physostigmine as to

Table II. Differential behavioral and neuroendocrine effects of physostigmine in affective-disorder patients and in patients with other psychiatric disorders [30]

Measure	Affective disorder patients		Other psychiatric patients	
	pre	post	pre	post
BPRS	n = 17		n = 20	
Depression	6.8 ± 0.4	12.4 ± 0.6	6.3 ± 0.4	8.5 ± 0.6*
Total	35.1 ± 2.0	48.9 ± 1.8	32.9 ± 1.4	38.5 ± 2.2*
A-I Scale				
Activation (rater)	9.4 ± 0.7	3.7 ± 0.8	9.2 ± 0.6	6.6 ± 0.7‡
Dysphoria (rater)	1.9 ± 0.5	5.6 ± 0.5	0.7 ± 0.2	2.3 ± 0.2‡
Inhibition (rater)	5.1 ± 1.3	31.4 ± 3.2	6.1 ± 1.7	17.6 ± 3.7†
Inhibition (subject)	18.4 ± 4.6	44.6 ± 4.1	14.9 ± 3.3	20.9 ± 3.3‡
POMS	n = 12		n = 18	
Tension-anxiety	14.0 ± 2.5	26.8 ± 2.4	8.4 ± 1.3	11.2 ± 1.6*
Depression-dejection	24.0 ± 5.1	36.0 ± 4.8	12.4 ± 3.1	13.7 ± 3.2 (p < 0.06)
Anger-hostility	13.4 ± 3.9	20.8 ± 3.3	5.7 ± 2.3	5.4 ± 1.8†
Fatigue	9.1 ± 3.0	19.0 ± 2.5	4.3 ± 1.3	8.7 ± 1.6‡
Friendliness	17.1 ± 2.6	9.8 ± 2.7	17.8 ± 1.8	15.4 ± 2.1‡

*p < 0.05; †p < 0.01; ‡p < 0.001.
(Originally published in Janowsky, Risch, Parker, et al., "Increased vulnerability to cholinergic stimulation in affect disorder patients," *Psychopharmacology Bulletin,* Vol. 16, No. 4, October 1980.)

development of behavioral inhibition and negative affect. Although this information could suggest that certain psychiatric patients, such as detoxified alcoholics, are hyporesponsive to cholinergic agents (i.e., they could have increased hepatic metabolism), the data also could indicate the existence of a relative or absolute cholinergic overactivity or receptor hypersensitivity in patients with major affective disorders. A normal control group is now being studied to confirm this differentiation.

Effects of Acetylcholine on Serum Growth Hormone, Prolactin and Cortisol

As part of the same study of the role of cholinergic factors in emotional disorders, we have studied the effects of physostigmine on several neurohormones, including prolactin, growth hormone, cortisol and luteinizing hormone [24]. The specific focus of this work has been to evaluate whether any of the above neurohormones change following infusion of physostigmine, and thus may serve as markers of physostigmine's effects.

Considerable evidence from animal experiments suggests that acetylcholine may play a role in neurohormone regulation. For example, cholinergic influences appear to play a part in modulating the control of the hypothalamic-pituitary axis.

The existence of a cholinergic link between the brain and the pituitary was suggested in early experiments in which gonadotropin secretion was modified by topical application of acetylcholine to the pituitary, and by the administration of cholinergic-blocking drugs to animals [25]. High doses of atropine [26], given intraventricularly, blocked ovulation and the peaks of LH, FSH, and prolactin that normally occur during the afternoon in proestrus rats, and also blocked the postgonadectomy rise of gonadotropin. The hypophysis of atropine-blocked rats liberated luteinizing hormone when the gland was adequately stimulated by LRF, indicating that atropine acts on the brain to modify the CNS control of the gland, rather than directly on the gland itself.

Although atropine inhibits the nocturnal surge and the proestrus prolactin surge in cycling rats [27], it is of interest that cholinergic agonists also may inhibit prolactin secretion [26]. However, in contrast, *Gibbs* et al. [28] have shown that intraventricular injection of acetylcholine in rats resulted in a marked increase of prolactin secretion which was not associated with an increase in the stalk dopamine levels.

In addition, cholinomimetic drugs have been shown in several studies, using isolated rat hypothalamic tissues, to release ACTH, although other studies in intact animals have not substantiated this finding [29].

On the basis of the above animal experiments, in experiments conducted at the University of California at San Diego over the past year, with methods essentially those described above, the influences of physostigmine on serum prolactin, growth hormone, and cortisol were studied [30]. Serum samples were obtained sequentially before and after placebo and physostigmine infusion and analyzed for serum prolactin, growth hormone, luteinizing hormone and cortisol using radioimmunoassay techniques. Overall, physostigmine, in contrast to placebo, caused significant increases in serum prolactin, cortisol, and growth hormone. In the small number of cases in which it was assayed, serum luteinizing hormone did not change. In addition, decrease in positive mood and increases in dysphoria and depression caused by physostigmine correlated negatively and positively, respectively, with serum prolactin changes. Increases in nausea correlated less dramatically, but significantly, with prolactin changes and the prolactin rise was twofold greater in patients with affect disorders. Serum cortisol increases after physostigmine showed no correlation with mood changes, nausea, or changes in serum prolactin or growth hormone. Serum growth hormone increases only infrequently correlated with mood changes.

These results concur with those of *Davis and Davis* [29] with respect to physostigmine's neurohormonal effects in man. Furthermore, our data suggest that the prolactin response may be a correlate of physostigmine's behavioral effects, and indeed may be a marker for patients with affect disorder. Whether the prolactin and cortisol response to physostigmine infusion is owing to specific acetylcholine hypothalamic effects or to nonspecific stress is an open question. However, the fact that the cortisol rise did not correlate with mood, diagnosis, or other neurohormone variables suggests a nonstress etiology.

Thus, serum prolactin and cortisol may be altered, in part, by cholinergic influences, and such effects may be specific rather than just caused by stress. Furthermore, if our observations concerning the effects of physostigmine on prolactin are owing to specific, rather than nonspecific effects, our data may indicate a dopamine system in patients with affect disorder which is vulnerable to inhibition by acetylcholine, since dopamine inhibits prolactin release. Alternatively, a cholinergic mechanism may be involved directly in the release of prolactin or cortisol.

Effects of Lithium on Cholinergic Function

Although the effects of lithium have been conceptualized as antiadrenergic and consistent with a catecholamine hypothesis of affective disorders [31], some findings from basic neurophysiology, reviewed elsewhere [32, 33], suggest that lithium may indeed affect central cholinergic processes.

In two experiments conducted by *Janowsky*, the interaction of lithium with the cholinergic nervous system was studied. In the first study [32], rats received physostigmine, physostigmine plus lithium (200 mg/kg for 4.5 days), or lithium plus physostigmine plus scopolamine. Lithium was found to increase physostigmine-induced lethality, an effect antagonized by scopolamine. These data suggest that acetylcholine activity or sensitivity might be enhanced by lithium. In contrast, in the other experiment [33], rats and mice were treated with methylphenidate followed by physostigmine or placebo. Animals were pretreated with either lithium or placebo for 7 days. Physostigmine, as observed previously [2], antagonized methylphenidate-induced gnawing behavior. Significantly, this effect was antagonized partially by lithium pretreatment. Thus, lithium appeared to antagonize a cholinergic effect.

In addition, *Jope* et al. [34] noted that red blood cell choline levels increase dramatically with lithium pretreatment. In preliminary studies, *Janowsky* et al. have also demonstrated that lithium pretreatment for 1–2 weeks indeed increases red blood cell choline levels. Our early results also indicate that titrated choline uptake into red blood cells is decreased following prior lithium treatment.

Since red blood cell choline utilization may reflect, in part, central processes and may determine acetylcholine synthesis and turnover, measurement of choline dynamics in red blood cells may give clues as to the pathophysiology of affective disorders. Our data so far suggest that, as in our lithium-physostigmine-methylphenidate animal behavioral experiment, lithium may decrease acetylcholine turnover.

Although lithium has been noted to decrease adrenergic activity and to antagonize some forms of psychostimulant-induced behavioral stimulation, and such findings have been used to support an antiadrenergic hypothesis for lithium's effects on mania, no satisfactory explanation of lithium's ameliorative effects on depression has yet been proposed. We have suggested that lithium's ability to antagonize the cholinergic effects of physostigmine may be an animal model of its ameliorative effects on depression in man [33]. We have postulated that lithium has a bidirectional effect on animal models of both mania and depression, based on its influence on adrenergic and cholinergic mechanisms, respectively. Lithium may, therefore, normalize the adrenergic and cholinergic nervous system of patients with affective disorders, antagonizing hypercholinergic and hyperadrenergic activity, and thus decreasing or preventing both depression and mania.

Conclusions

This review indirectly suggests a role for cholinergic mechanisms in the regulation and, possibly, the etiology of affective disorders. However, it is important to note that, as with all biologic hypotheses of affective disorders, evidence contradicting this hypothesis does exist. First, and most important, although anticholinergic agents have been reported to cause euphoria in some patients, they are not particularly good antidepressants. Second, although most tricyclic antidepressants have anticholinergic (antimuscarinic) properties, they do not universally have these properties in equal amounts, and their potency is not particularly linked to antimuscarinic activity [35]. It is important, however, to note that the ability of chronically administered antidepressants to reduce acetylcholine activity has not been studied as such. Furthermore, the dramatic effects on mood of such acetylcholinesterase inhibitors as physostigmine indicate that in some way, either directly or indirectly (i.e., by affecting norepinephrine, dopamine, GABA, or other neuromodulators), acetylcholine is quite likely to be involved in the regulation of affect and in the pathophysiology of affective disorders.

Acknowledgment

This research was supported in part by NIMH grant No. 5 P50 MH 30914-04.

References

1   Janowsky, D.S.; El-Yousef, M.K.; Davis, J.M.; et al.: A cholinergic-adrenergic hypothesis of mania and depression. Lancet *ii:* 632–635 (1972).
2   Janowsky, D.S.; El-Yousef, M.K.; Davis, J.M.; et al.: Cholinergic antagonism of methylphenidate-induced stereotyped behavior. Psychopharmacologia *27:* 295–303 (1972).
3   Janowsky, D.S.; El-Yousef, M.K.; Davis, J.M.; et al.: Parasympathetic suppression of manic symptoms by physostigmine. Archs. gen. Psychiat. *28:* 542–547 (1973).
4   Goodman, L.S.; Gilman, A.: in The pharmacological basis of therapeutics; 4th ed. (Collier-Macmillan, Toronto 1970).
5   Rowntree, D.W.; Neven, S.; Wilson, A.: The effects of diisopropylfluorophosphonate in schizophrenia and manic depressive psychosis. J. Neurol. Neurosurg. Psychiat. *13:* 47–62 (1950).
6   Gershon, S.; Shaw, F.H.: Psychiatric sequelae of chronic exposure to organophosphorous insecticides. Lancet *i:* 1371–1374 (1961).
7   Bowers, M.B.; Goodman, E.; Sim, V.M.: Some behavioral changes in man following anticholinesterase administration. J. Nerv. Ment. Dis. *138:* 383 (1964).
8   Janowsky, D.S.; Davis, J.M.; El-Yousef, M.K.; et al.: Acetylcholine and depression. Psychosom. Med. *35:* 568 (1973).
9   Modestin, J.J.; Schwartz, R.B.; Hunger, J.: Zur Frage der Beeinflussung schizophrener Symptome durch Physostigmin. Pharmakopsychiatrie *9:* 300–304 (1973).
10 Modestin, J.J.; Hunger, R.B.; Schwartz, R.B.: Über die depressogene Wirkung von Physostigmin. Arch. Psychiat. NervKr. ankh. *218:* 67 (1973).
11 Carroll, B.J.; Frazer, A.; Schless, A.; et al.: Cholinergic reversal of manic symptoms. Lancet *i:* 427 (1973).
12 Davis, K.L.; Berger, P.A.; Hollister, L.E.; et al.: Physostigmine in mania. Archs. gen. Psychiat. *35:* 119–122 (1978).
13 Shopsin, B.; Janowsky, D.S.; Davis, J.M.; et al.: Rebound phenomena in manic patients following physostigmine. Neuropsychobiology *1:* 180–187 (1975).
14 El-Yousef, M.K.; Janowsky, D.S.; Davis, J.M.; et al.: Induction of severe

depression by physostigmine in marijuana-intoxicated individuals. Br. J. Addict. 68: 321–325 (1973).

15 Rosenblatt, J.E.; Janowsky, D.S.; Davis, J.M.; et al.: The augmentation of physostigmine toxicity in the rat by delta-9-tetrahydrocannabinol. Res. Commun. chem. Pathol. Pharm. 3: 479–482 (1972).

16 Davis, K. L.; Hollister, L.E.; Overall, J.; et al.: Physostigmine. Effects on cognition and affect in normal subjects. Psychopharmacology 51: 23–27 (1976).

17 Tamminga, C.; Smith, R.C.; Chang, S.; et al.: Depression associated with oral choline. Lancet ii: 905 (1976).

18 Davis, K.: Effects of choline in schizophrenia. Am. J. Psychiat. (in press, 1980).

19 Casey, D.E.: Mood alterations during deanol therapy. Psychopharmacology 62· 187–191 (1979).

20 Sitarm, N.; Nurnberger, J.I.; Gershon, E.; et al.: Faster REM sleep induction in euthymic patients with preliminary affective illness. Science 208: 200–202 (1980).

21 Kupfer, D.J.; Foster, F.G.; Reich, L.; et al.: EEG sleep changes as predictors in depression. Am. J. Psychiat. 133: 622–626 (1976).

22 Carroll, B.J.; Greden, J.F.; Rubin, R.T.; et al.: Neurotransmitter mechanism of neuro-endocrine disturbance in depression. Acta endocr., Copenh., 220, suppl., p. 14 (1978).

23 Oppenheimer, G.; Ebstein, R.; Belmaker, R.: Effect of lithium on the physostigmine-induced behavioral syndrome and plasma cyclic GMP. J. psychiat. Res. 14: 133–138 (1979).

24 Janowsky, E.S.; Risch, S.C.; Judd, L.L.; et al.: Acetylcholine sensitivity in affect disorders. Ann. Meet. Am. Psychiat. Ass., San Francisco 1980.

25 Everett, J.W.: Central neural control of reproductive functions of the adenohypophysis. Physiol. Rev. 44: 373 (1964).

26 Libertun, C.; McCann, S.M.: Blockade of the release of gonadotropin and prolactin by subcutaneous or intraventricular injection of atropine in male and female rats. Endocrinology 92: 1714 (1973).

27 Libertun, C.; McCann, S.M.: Further evidence for cholinergic control of gonadotropin and prolactin secretion. Proc. Soc. exp. Biol. Med. 147: 498 (1974).

28 Gibbs, D.M.; Plotsky, P.M.; de Greff, W.J.; et al.: Effect of histamine and acetylcholine on hypophyseal stalk plasma dopamine and peripheral plasma prolactin levels. Life Sci. 24: 2063–2070 (1979).

29 Davis, K.L.; Davis, B.M.: Acetylcholine and anterior pituitary hormone secretion; in Davis, Berger, Brain acetylcholine and neuropsychiatric disease (Plenum Press, New York 1979).

30 Janowsky, D.S.; Risch, S.C.; Parker, D.; et al.: Increased vulnerability to cholinergic stimulation in affect disorder patients. Psychopharmacol. Bull. 16 (4) (1980).

31 Ebstein, R.; Belmaker, R.H.; Grinhaus: Lithium inhibition of adrenaline-stimulated adenylate cyclase in humans. Nature, Lond. 249: 411 (1976).

32 Samples, J.; Janowsky, D.S.; Pechnick, R.; et al.: Lethal effects of physostigmine plus lithium in rats. Psychopharmacology 52: 307–309 (1977).

33 Janowsky, D.S.; Abrams, A.; Judd, L.L.; et al.: Lithium administration antago-

| 34 | Jope, R.S.; Jenden, D.J.; Erlich, B.E.: Choline accumulates in erythrocytes during lithium therapy. New Engl. J. Med. *299:* 833–834 (1978). |
| 35 | Snyder, S.H.; Yamamura, H.I.: Antidepressants and the muscarinic acetylcholine receptor. Archs. gen. Psychiat. *34:* 236–239 (1977). |

nizes cholinergic behavioral effects in rodents. Psychopharmacology *63:* 147–150 (1979).

Discussion

Mendels: We have to look at new data in context and not make more of them than is appropriate. There are data, for instance, about giving physostigmine to manics and altering their mood state; and then there are other data about altering the mood state in actual unipolar or bipolar depressed patients. A problem with the marijuana studies is that there is a different chemical state to start with. The question which I have is: to what extent are alcoholics appropriate for control studies, or candidates for any affect disorder study?

Janowsky: Other than that they have some chemical toxicity, why wouldn't they be?

Mendels: Besides liver alterations, who knows what damage or alterations have occurred in the brain, or what possible genetic associations and links there may be? There are a number of reasons why I would be a little cautious about comparing groups containing alcoholics.

Janowsky: You are right. However, even with normal subjects you can come up with similar kinds of issues: a normal person who is not an inpatient or did not have the same experiences, and so on. With any form of research, somebody will look at your results from another point of view. In the end, there may be an answer that will fit.

Maas: If you have a patient who comes in with an overdose of a tricyclic, do you use physostigmine? What are the indications for its use? What dosage do you use?

Janowsky: Physostigmine is overused in my opinion. In the case of overdoses of tricyclics, many patients will get groggy or confused. Sometimes they will have a tricyclic central anticholinergic confusional state. It may last a day or two. If you can wait, patients will clear up in a day or two, unless it is a massive overdose. If the patient is uncontrollable, you might want to use physostigmine. If you do use it, you should give approximately 2 mg or more, either intramuscularly or intravenously every 2 h as physostigmine has a short half-life. You have to continue monitoring the patient and be sure that the patient continues to receive physostigmine.

Neuroendocrine Aspects of Depression: Theoretical and Practical Significance

Bernard J. Carroll

Clinical Studies Unit; Mental Health Research Institute, University of Michigan, Ann Arbor, Michigan

Origins of the Neuroendocrine Strategy

The neuroendocrine approach to research in depression provides a functional system for testing neurotransmitter theories, such as the monoamine theory of depression. Also, in principle, study of the neuroendocrine system allows assessment of the integrity of limbic system nuclei in the brains of patients with psychopathology. Perhaps equally important to investigators is the opportunity to evaluate the action of drugs on neuroendocrine systems, as evidenced, for example, by the widely known elevation of prolactin secretion by neuroleptics. In depression, specifically, neuroendocrine indices may be used to test theories about the mode of action of antidepressant drugs.

The rationale for the neuroendocrine approach is illustrated in figure 1, which gives a schematic outline of the neuroendocrine system. The importance of the limbic system nuclei above the hypothalamic median eminence level is well illustrated here. The cortical and subcortical regions of the limbic system (such as hippocampus, amygdala, frontal cortex, temporal cortex, parts of midbrain, and septal nuclei) communicate by synaptic neurotransmitter links with the median eminence and hypothalamus. The fine tuning of neuroendocrine regulation, including circadian rhythms and responses to stress, comes from these inputs. It is important to note that these neurotransmitter links with the hypothalamus are especially vulnerable to spontaneous disturbances, such as depression and drug effects.

The remaining steps in the neuroendocrine cascade are more strictly endocrine in nature. The median eminence and hypothalamic neurons secrete the so-called releasing and inhibiting hormones into the pituitary portal vascular system, by which route they reach the anterior pituitary. The hypothalamic hor-

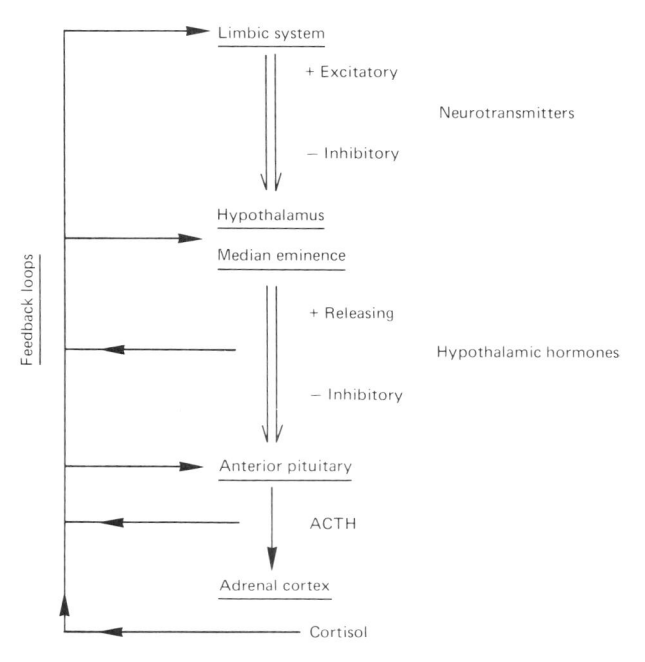

Fig. 1. Basic organization of neuroendocrine systems, illustrated by the ACTH-cortisol system.

mones then stimulate or inhibit the synthesis and release of pituitary hormones into the general circulation. The next step in the cascade is the release of peripheral hormones, such as cortisol, by ACTH. Finally, both the peripheral and pituitary hormones can exert feedback effects on the pituitary, hypothalamic, or limbic system sites.

Most of the reliable information that has emerged from the neuroendocrine approach to the study of depression reflects the possibility that a disturbance at the highest level of the neuroendocrine systems has led to the illness. This disturbance may involve, for example, synaptic relays between the limbic system and the hypothalamus. Recent studies of hypothalamic hormones suggest that functional relationships at the second level of the system also may be abnormal, but much of the evidence in this area is preliminary [6].

ACTH-Cortisol System in Depression

It has been well documented that cortisol production is excessive in about 50% of patients with depression [3]. As clinical neuroendocrine techniques have been developed, the true nature of cortisol hypersecretion by depressed patients has been determined. Plasma cortisol levels show their greatest elevation above control values during the late afternoon and evening hours, and during the early hours of sleep [8], not during the early part of the day (8–10 A.M.). In many cases, there is apparently a phase advance of 1–2 h in the onset of the major circadian secretory episode of cortisol [8]. Thus, in depressed patients, this early morning secretion of cortisol may begin at about 2–3 A.M. rather than at 3–5 A.M. Moreover, depressed patients frequently do not manifest the normal spontaneous inhibition of cortisol secretion during the evening hours. Rather, they continue to show disinhibited secretion of cortisol that is inappropriate for this phase of the circadian cycle [8]. Even during sleep, the disinhibited hypersecretion of cortisol may persist in these patients and is not related to the occurrence of dreaming rapid eye movement (REM) episodes [8]. Evidence such as this has helped establish that the increased cortisol secretion of depressed patients is not simply a result of the distress they are experiencing. Rather, their disinhibited secretion of cortisol now is regarded as a reflection of a disturbed limbic system function. In this regard, it must be recalled that the limbic system of the brain regulates neuroendocrine function as well as emotional or affective functions and the autonomic nervous system.

The hypersecretion of cortisol in depression has been characterized in many converging ways. These patients frequently will show elevated 24-hour secretion rates of cortisol and high values for urinary cortisol metabolite excretion, such as 17-OHCS or 17-KGS [2]. The tissue exposure to physiologically active cortisol also is increased as reflected by urinary free cortisol (UFC) excretion [3]. Direct measurements of free, nonprotein-bound cortisol in plasma and cerebrospinal fluid confirm this conclusion [3]. By all of these indices, patients with severe depression may show hypersecretion of cortisol to an extent observed in some patients with Cushing's disease. Indeed, Cushing's disease with associated depression may sometimes be difficult to differentiate diagnostically from depression with Cushing-like hypersecretion of cortisol. In general, however, patients with primary depression will not manifest the peripheral signs of hypercortisolism that are so characteristic of Cushing's disease, although their depression may be of many months' duration.

Some dynamic tests of neuroendocrine regulation in depressed patients give results that are similar to those seen in Cushing's disease. These include both stimulatory and suppressive test procedures. For example, the cortisol and growth hormone (GH) responses to insulin-induced hypoglycemia are blunted in depressed patients as they are in diencephalic Cushing's disease [3]. These findings should be interpreted with some caution, however, since in many studies depressed patients have been found to be somewhat resistant to the hypoglycemic action of insulin. Consequently, they have not always achieved an adequate degree or duration of hypoglycemia to generate a normal cortisol or GH response. Since the physiologic stimulus of hypoglycemia can be difficult to standardize between patients (or between tests within the same patient), the insulin-induced hypoglycemia test is not widely used now for the evaluation of subtle neuroendocrine disturbances in depression.

Suppression of cortisol secretion by dexamethasone is another dynamic aspect of hypothalamic-pituitary-adrenal (HPA) function that has been studied extensively, using several different regimens of dexamethasone administration. In all the studies, some depressed patients have been identified who have failed to suppress cortisol secretion normally [5]. For example, even with an extended high-dosage dexamethasone regimen (2 mg every 6 h for 48 h), failure of normal suppression to dexamethasone has been observed in depressed patients. This is highly significant since, ordinarily, only patients with severe Cushing's disease or Cushing's syndrome would fail to suppress with this dosage of dexamethasone.

In the dexamethasone suppression test (DST), synthetic glucocorticoid (dexamethasone) substitutes for the natural cortisol in the feedback loop at the level of the pituitary gland. Dexamethasone also has a minor effect on the fast-feedback action of cortisol at the median eminence level. Dexamethasone, however, does not bind to glucocorticoid receptors for cortisol in the limbic regions of the brain. By flooding glucocorticoid receptors in the anterior pituitary, dexamethasone causes a decrease in ACTH secretion. This leads, in turn, to a lowering of cortisol secretion. For this action of dexamethasone to be impaired, it is thought that an excessive release of the stimulatory hypothalamic hormone for ACTH (corticotropin-releasing factor) must occur, both in severe depression and in Cushing's disease of diencephalic origin. One other possibility that cannot be excluded yet is that such patients have abnormal glucocorticoid receptor binding of dexamethasone by the anterior pituitary. It has been established, however, that the metabolism and circulating plasma levels of dexamethasone are quite normal in those depressed patients who fail to show normal suppression of plasma cortisol after dexamethasone. Thus, the discovery of abnormal DST results indicates that some type of central neuroendocrine disturbance is present.

The most widely used regimen of dexamethasone administration in research studies of depression is the overnight DST procedure. Dexamethasone is given at 11–12 P.M., and blood samples for plasma cortisol are drawn the following day. This regimen was first introduced by clinical endocrinologists as a screening test for Cushing's disease, and a single blood sample at 8 A.M. was regarded generally as sufficient to evaluate the suppression response. More recently, it has been found that normal subjects will maintain suppression of plasma cortisol for at least 24 h after 1-2 mg dexamethasone given at 12 P.M. [5]. Frequent sampling catheter studies have shown, further, that depressed patients often have an abnormal, early escape of plasma cortisol levels rather than an absolute resistance to suppression by dexamethasone [5]. In this respect, the disinhibition of HPA activity in depressed patients usually is less severe than that seen in Cushing's disease. Nonetheless, when compared with normal subjects, depressed patients show a definite, though subtle, neuroendocrine disturbance.

The standard DST protocol now used for inpatients calls for three blood samples at 8 A.M., 4 P.M., and 11 P.M. after oral administration of 1 mg dexamethasone at 11 P.M. the preceding night. For outpatients, a practical compromise is to obtain only one postdexamethasone blood sample at 4 P.M. Based on inpatient studies, about 80% of the abnormal DST results will be detected at 4 P.M. by this sample. The criterion of a normal DST response is that all plasma cortisol levels should be less than 5 μg/dl after administration of dexamethasone. An abnormal DST response in depression is manifested typically as an escape of plasma cortisol levels by 4 P.M., following temporary suppression at 8 A.M. The escape may occur less commonly by 8 A.M., or not until between 4 and 11 P.M. In early studies with the DST, the postdexamethasone UFC excretion was evaluated as an index of the HPA suppression response [2]. Since the urinary measure was later found to give only a small amount of additional information, it has been eliminated from the current test protocol. As a result, the DST procedure now not only is standardized but is also extremely simple for inpatient and outpatient use.

Clinical Studies with the DST

Relation to Episodes
When abnormal DST results indicative of disinhibited HPA activity occur in depressed patients, they are closely linked to the actual episode of illness. In fact, when the patient has recovered, normal DST responses will be found [2]. Thus, the DST cannot be used to help detect a tendency toward depression in asymptomatic persons, such as family members at risk for the illness. If an abnormal DST response fails to convert to normal with treatment, despite apparent clinical improvement, the patient will be at high risk for early relapse [2]. In the few cases that have been studied by the DST at frequent intervals during

treatment, a gradual improvement of the neuroendocrine response has been seen as the patients improved clinically [2]. A small number of rapidly cycling bipolar depressives have been studied during the switch process into depression, and it has been observed that abnormal DST results may precede the clinical change by 24–48 h. Such observations suggest that if a neuroendocrine disturbance is seen, it reflects the underlying pathology of the illness within the limbic system.

Relation to Polarity

Abnormal DST results have been described with approximately equal frequency in both bipolar and unipolar endogenous depressive patients. When bipolar patients are in a manic or hypomanic phase of illness, the DST responses are normal. This finding indicates that mania is a distinctly different state from depression, at least with respect to this particular neuroendocrine marker. It contradicts the so-called continuum theories, which claim that mania is fundamentally the same disorder as depression, only more severe.

Specificity

The abnormal DST responses found in unipolar and bipolar endogenous depressives are rarely seen in normal subjects or in other psychiatric patients. It is important to keep in mind the distinction between endogenous and nonendogenous (neurotic or reactive) depression when reports of the DST are being evaluated. Patients with nonendogenous depression, like normal subjects, have a low frequency of abnormal DST response (less than 5%) [3]. Similarly, patients with most other psychiatric disorders have the same low frequency of abnormal DST results [1, 9].

On the other hand, diurnal or nocturnal measures of baseline (spontaneous) hypersecretion of cortisol do not distinguish as clearly endogenous depressives from other types of patients [3]. The DST appears to achieve its high specificity by eliminating the nonspecific secretion of cortisol associated with psychologic distress. A more specific form of limbic system activation or disinhibition is needed to overcome the HPA-suppressing action of dexamethasone.

Sensitivity

Only 50%, approximately, of patients with unipolar or bipolar endogenous depression have disinhibited HPA activity or abnormal DST responses. A summary of recent studies with the DST from Michigan, Rhode Island, and Iowa City [9] indicates that the overall sensitivity of this test was about 45% among nearly 200 patients. In the same studies, the overall specificity was 98% among nearly 200 comparison patients.

Diagnostic Utility

Based on the sensitivity and specificity results described, it now is possible to use the DST for diagnostic purposes. The diagnostic confidence or predictive value associated with a positive DST result is better than 95%. Thus, a positive DST result may be used with some real confidence to support the diagnosis of endogenous depression. The test can be especially useful in cases where a mixture of endogenous or reactive features leads to diagnostic uncertainty, or where an atypical presentation, such as catatonia, occurs.

On the other hand, a negative DST result does not necessarily rule out the diagnosis of endogenous depression since only about 45% of patients with this diagnosis are identified by the test. Thus, a negative or normal DST result is less informative than a positive result. To improve the rate of positive identification of both endogenous and nonendogenous cases, other supplemental laboratory procedures are needed.

Certain technical factors also need to be kept in mind if the DST is to be used for diagnostic purposes. Patients with endocrine disease must be excluded as well as patients receiving high-dosage estrogens. Severe weight loss (to below 80% of ideal body weight), as occurs in malnutrition or anorexia nervosa, is associated with a false-positive DST results. Similarly, patients with severe systemic medical conditions, fever, and/or dehydration, must be excluded. Finally, certain drugs accelerate the hepatic metabolism of dexamethasone including anticonvulsants or relaxants, such as phenytoin, phenobarbital, other barbiturates, and meprobamate. Patients who have taken them within the past 3 weeks must be excluded.

Heterogeneity

It is clear that a subgroup of patients with endogenous depression have a specific neuroendocrine disturbance of disinhibited HPA activity. A distinctive clinical profile of this subgroup has not emerged, however, so that clinical features cannot be used to predict which patients with endogenous depression will have an abnormal DST response. Neither has any particular association between DST response and treatment response been observed. The heterogeneity among endogenous depressives with respect to this neuroendocrine marker is so far unexplained. One group of investigators has suggested that genetic factors may account for the heterogeneity, but this report has not yet been confirmed [9].

Etiologic Significance

The studies of HPA function carried out so far do not give a definite answer about the etiologic significance of the neuroendocrine disturbances identified in depressed patients. While there is definitely a close time relationship between depressive episodes and HPA disinhibition, the heterogeneity and lack of association with treatment outcome, even among definite bipolar depressives, raise the possibility that the neuroendocrine disturbances are epiphenomena. Thus, they may be related to the primary limbic-system etiology in an inconstant and indirect way. In other words, the neuroendocrine disturbances may reflect limbic system noise associated with depressive episodes. This need not detract, however, from the practical diagnostic usefulness of the neuroendocrine markers, such as the DST.

The neurotransmitter mechanism of the neuroendocrine disturbances is also being investigated. In the case of the CRF-ACTH-cortisol system, a muscarinic cholinergic mechanism has been identified by which escape from dexamethasone suppression can occur. From animal studies, however, it is clear that several neurotransmitters interact in the regulation of this system. These include acetylcholine, norepinephrine, serotonin, GABA, and possibly the opioid peptide system as well.

Until the actions and interactions of these various neurotransmitters are identified in human subjects and in depressed patients, it will not be possible to use the neuroendocrine findings as outright support for the various neurotransmitter theories of depression. The hope remains, nonetheless, that future studies will show the neuroendocrine changes to be mediated by the same neurotransmitter pathologic process as the illness itself. If this is confirmed, then investigators will have a powerful means of studying in vivo the neurochemical mechanisms of depression as well as the action of antidepressant therapeutic agents.

Discussion

Research studies of the HPA system have shown that neuroendocrine disinhibition occurs in about 50% of patients with endogenous depression. The overall pattern of disturbances in endogenous depression is similar to that seen in diencephalic Cushing's disease. The best documented and most specific measure of disinhibited HPA activity is the dexamethasone suppression test. Results obtained in several centers with this test indicate that a positive test result may be used with a high degree of confidence to support a diagnosis of endogenous depression. A negative result, on the other hand, does not necessarily rule out the diagnosis of endogenous depression. The disinhibited HPA activity is closely related in time to episodes of depression and may be a reflection of limbic system "noise" in depressed patients. The neuroendocrine heterogeneity of endogenous depressives and the neurotransmitter mechanisms of the HPA disinhibition are currently being studied in the hope that they will lead to an understanding of the basic mechanisms of depression.

References

1   Brown, W.A.; Johnson, R.; Mayfield, D.: The 24-hour dexamethasone suppression test in a clinical setting: relationship to diagnosis, symptoms and response to treatment. Am. J. Psychiat. *136:* 543–547 (1979).
2   Carroll, B.J.: The hypothalamic-pituitary-adrenal axis in depression; in Davies, Carroll, Mowbray, Depressive illness: some research studies (Thomas, Springfield 1972).
3   Carroll, B.J.: Neuroendocrine function in psychiatric disorders; in Lipton, DiMascio, Killam, Psychopharmacology: a generation of progress. (Raven Press, New York 1978).
4   Carroll, B.J.: Implications of biological research for the diagnosis of depression; in Mendlewicz, New advances in the diagnosis and treatment of depressive illness (Elsevier, Amsterdam, in press, 1980).
5   Carroll, B.J.; Mendels, J.: Neuroendocrine regulation in affective disorders; in Sachar, Hormones, behavior and psychopathology (Raven Press, New York 1976).
6   Ettigi, P.G.; Brown, G.M.: Psychoneuroendocrinology of affective disorders: an overview. Am. J. Psychiat. *134:* 493–501 (1977).
7   Sachar, E.J.: ACTH and cortisol secretion in psychiatric disease; in Krieger, Ganong, ACTH and related peptides: structure, regulation and action, pp. 621–627 (Academic Press, New York 1977).
8   Sachar, E.J.; Hellman, L.; Roffwarg, H.; et al.: Disrupted 24-hour patterns of cortisol secretion in psychotic depression. Archs. gen. Psychiat. *28:* 19–24 (1973).
9   Schlesser, M.A.; Winokur, G.; Sherman, B.M.: Genetic subtypes of unipolar primary depressive illness distinguished by hypothalamic-pituitary-adrenal axis activity. Lancet *i:* 739–741 (1979).

Discussion

Katz: What is the relationship, in your judgment, between nonendogenous and endogenous depressions and severity of depression? Also, presumably the only characteristic of the RDC that distinguishes it from other diagnostic systems is that the RDC standardizes criteria so that we know what the clinician means when he refers to a particular type of affective disorder. What is your opinion?

Carroll: It's not related. The mean Hamilton and mean self-rating scores of nonendogenous cases were not different from all the endogenous cases. The mean Hamilton score was 18.6 for the endogenous cases and 16.6 for the nonendogenous cases; the mean self-ratings were 23.4 and 23.5, respectively. When you use the Hamilton scale with the Newcastle Index, for example, you can't identify a severity difference between endogenous and nonendogenous cases.

To answer your other question, there are two areas of diagnostic disagreement. One is between the clinical diagnosis of endogenous depression and the RDC diagnosis of major depressive disorder. That's easy to handle because it's essentially a definitional difference. The criteria for endogenous depression are different from the much looser entry criteria for major depressive disorders. Our own criteria for endogenous depression include the RDC criteria for endogenous depression and also incorporation of a history of episodes, family history, bipolar course, and previous treatment response. These are items that clinicians generally weigh heavily but which are not included in the RDC.

The second source of disagreement in diagnoses is where the clinicians feel a patient does not have an endogenous depression, but according to the RDC it is. If we follow strictly the literal operational RDC guidelines, then patients will often qualify for a number of items that the clinicians will discount.

Secunda: If I, for example, give a patient 1 mg of dexamethasone, draw the blood and ship it off to a lab, will I get a reliable cortisol reading back? Can clinicians make practical use of an outside laboratory in this way?

Carroll: I would talk with the laboratory technician before I did that, but in principle the answer is yes.

Mendels: The average psychiatrists are not in a position to talk to the laboratory personnel, and if they do, they may not know what to say and what questions to ask.

Carroll: They should ask the laboratory director if they have high precision tests in the low value range for cortisol so that a value of 6 can be discriminated from 4 or 3, for example, or if the assay is geared more toward picking up values in the 20-30 range, as when endocrinologists look at patients with Cushing's disease. Some laboratories will not normally discriminate between values below 5, for example, but they will do that if you ask them.

Secunda: Most psychiatrists do not routinely take blood. Is this a problem?

Carroll: No. You just send patients to a clinical laboratory if you do not feel comfortable drawing blood.

Dunner: It's important to underscore the fact that the dexamethasone test is state-dependent. It may be that some of the differences in results are related somehow to severity of illness in the outpatient population. Also, I assume that there is diagnostic agreement that the bipolar patients you had were endogenomorphic, or RDC-positive, which then underscores the lack of diagnostic agreement on the rest of the unipolar disorders.

Carroll: Right. The disagreements were all with unipolar patients.

Lipton: For the sake of the practitioner, again, of the 17 patients who were severely depressed and had normal responses to dexamethasone suppression, two-thirds showed a poor response to tricyclics. How would you treat them?

Carroll: They were finally treated with ECT.

Lipton: Did they respond well?

Carroll: Finally.

Mendels: Are you saying that patients with endogenous depression did not respond to tricyclics?

Carroll: Yes, but they later responded to ECT.

Hawkins: What is the real advantage for the clinician of doing the dexamethasone test unless you are assuming that he's not a skilled diagnostician?

Carroll: This is a very important point. The highest frequency of abnormal responses occurs where clinicians are most sure; where the clinicians are doubtful, the frequency is somewhat lower, about 20%. So, in a sense, the increase in risk ratio for the diagnosis is not greatly increased in the probable group by using the test. Where we have found the test helpful to the average clinician is where the presentations are atypical, such as in catatonic patients, or where the patient has a mild depression in the context of some situational and reactive factors. In such cases there is often diagnostic disagreement among clinicians as to the best way to treat these patients. Some physicians are focusing on the psychologic problems, and others believe that this is an endogenous depression despite the apparent psychogenic problems. In such cases, the dexamethasone test has proved invaluable to us. When a positive result was obtained, we followed that patient during treatment and found that the diagnosis of endogenous depression was correct.

Mendels: Another possible advantage is the ability to verify a diagnosis. A skilled clinical endocrinologist may feel able to diagnose hypothyroidism clinically and yet wouldn't be satisfied without tests to verify his clinical diagnosis. If this test covers 50% of patients, it seems to me that it's a step in the direction which many of us would like clinical psychiatrists take. It provides another way of approaching patients in a more systematic manner. The test is relatively simple and nonintrusive. That may be as important as the number of occasional patients whom you might otherwise misdiagnose.

Carroll: It is a good point. If I may use another analogy, hematologists can treat anemia by looking at the patient's eyelids, but they wouldn't. If you believe that this neuroendocrine disturbance has constructive validity for the endogenous depressions, then it's worth using as a marker. The other payoff is that it can be used to confirm that the episode is terminated.

Hawkins: Don't we require other markers that are more practical tests for common clinical use?

Carroll: We are now combining this test with one of the growth hormone procedures, the amphetamine response, and also with the sleep EEG. We have preliminary data with the growth hormone test in 10 patients who had a negative dexamethasone test result. They then had the amphetamine-stimulated growth hormone test. Five patients diagnosed as nonendogenous or neurotic by the clinicians had a normal growth hormone response consistent with neurotic status or with nonendogenous status, whereas three of the five patients diagnosed as having endogenous depression had an inadequate growth hormone response consistent with previous reports. If these data hold up, 80% of the variance in the dexamethasone-negative group may be cleared up by adding the second test. The hope is that we can get a positive laboratory identification of endogenous versus nonendogenous depression in upwards of 85% of patients by using both tests.

The Psychobiology of Affective Disorders. Pfizer Symp. Depression, Boca Raton 1980, pp. 111–129 (Karger, Basel 1980)

Effect of Tricyclic Antidepressants on Cerebral Capillary Permeability: An Action on a Fundamental Cerebral Homeostatic Mechanism

Boyd K. Hartman*
Washington University School of Medicine, St. Louis, Missouri

Introduction

The central adrenergic system has been implicated in the mediation of a seemingly endless variety of normal and abnormal physiologic functions and behavioral states. These include eating and drinking behavior, temperature regulation, sleep, aggression, stress, motivation, alertness, attention, and rage, as well as psychiatric affective disorders, such as schizophrenia and alcoholism. It is even more remarkable when one considers that the neurons within the brain containing norepinephrine or epinephrine number in the tens of thousands, compared with the other types of neurons which number in the billions.

Many investigators might argue about the strength of the evidence supporting catecholamine mediation of many of the phenomena listed. Few would deny, however, that alterations in central catecholamine metabolism can be measured in a wide variety of physiologic or pharmacologic states. A number of conceptual frameworks have been proposed in an attempt to tie together under some unifying principle these diverse potential functions. The framework most familiar to psychiatrists emphasizes the adrenergic efferent connections to the limbic forebrain. This portion of the brain is phylogenetically old and is thought to be important in intensely emotional states. While this concept may explain some manifestations of depression, the largest portion of the central adrenergic system which is not associated with the limbic system is ignored.

Some investigators have emphasized the adrenergic connections involving various brain regions known to regulate hormone release (for example, the

---

*In association with S.H. Preskorn, M.E. Raichle, L.W. Swanson and H.B. Clark supraoptic and paraventricular nuclei whose cells produce oxytocin and vasopressin), or influence blood pressure (for example, the vagal complex and the preganglionic sympathetic neurons of the intermedial lateral cell column of the spinal cord). Still others have investigated the effect of the system on the electrophysiologic state of individual neurons. Although frequently results appeared inconsistent, it gradually became clear that the specific effect of norepinephrine on the excitability of a given cell is dependent on the electrophysiologic state of the cell at the time of synaptic release. Thus, the central adrenergic system can be viewed as a regulatory system capable of enhancing specific signals while at the same time dampening others, depending on the specific needs of the organism at the time. This concept explains many aspects of the system. However, it does not take into account evidence of another important function of the central adrenergic system, i.e., the innervation of nonneuronal elements such as blood vessels and glial cells.

The purpose of this paper is to present evidence for an additional concept, viewing the central adrenergic system as part of an intra-axial autonomic system. Its function is to provide autonomic control for the brain analogous to that which the remainder of the body receives from the sympathetic nervous system. In addition, our evidence will show that a complete understanding of the pharmacologic action of tricyclic antidepressants must take into account microvascular effects mediated by the central adrenergic system.

Anatomical Similarities between the Central Adrenergic and Peripheral Adrenergic (Sympathetic) Neuron Systems

Our original hypothesis, that the functions of the central and peripheral adrenergic systems might be similar, was based on the similarity of the anatomical organization of these two adrenergic systems [1]. The cell bodies of both systems are clustered together in well-defined groups. In the peripheral system, these groups of cell bodies are, of course, the various sympathetic ganglia. In the brain, the groups of adrenergic cell bodies are designated by numbers A1–A7 in a more or less caudal to rostral sequence. *Dahlström and Fuxe* [2] first described these cell bodies. The largest single group is the locus ceruleus. It is located just lateral to the fourth ventricle in the pons. The axon systems of both central and peripheral neurons also have many features in common. They are generally long, small in diameter and unmyelinated. The axons are also highly branched. This allows for a remarkably divergent system. Thus, input into the superior cervical sympathetic ganglion can influence structures as distant and dissimilar as the pial vasculature of the brain, the iris, and the salivary glands. Similarly, in the brain, input to the locus ceruleus may influence such divergent brain areas as the cerebellum, the hippocampus, the cerebral cortex, neurosecretion in the paraventricular nucleus, transmission of visual impulses through the lateral geniculate body, and auditory impulses through the cochlear nucleus.

The axons in both systems undergo final branching to form plexuses of varicosed fibers in the innervated regions. Transmitter release in both systems apparently occurs at these varicosities. Similarities are present in the innervated structures, although their differences are emphasized more often. In the periphery, one usually thinks of innervation of nonneuronal elements, blood vessels, glands, etc. It should not be forgotten, however, that peripheral neurons also receive sympathetic innervation (e.g., neurons of the myenteric plexuses). In the brain, one thinks of interactions with other neurons. There is strong evidence, however, that nonneuronal elements in the brain are also innervated by the central adrenergic system. One of the early observations using dopamine-beta-hydroxylase (DBH) as a marker for the central adrenergic system showed the frequent, close association of the central adrenergic fibers with cerebral microvessels [1, 3, 4]. Direct contact of adrenergic terminals with the capillary endothelium has been demonstrated at the electron microscopic level [5]. This is not to suggest that the central adrenergic system does not specifically interact with other neurons. There is no question that synaptic interactions with central neurons exist. In some regions, 20% or more of the varicosities may be involved in specialized synaptic contacts with other neurons. However, in some brain regions, as few as 5% of the varicosities have been reported to exhibit synaptic contacts. Losing sight of the nonneuronal interactions may obscure the basic autonomic nature of the system.

A general description of the anatomical organization of the central adrenergic system would necessarily include both types of innervation. A widespread and diffuse plexus of varicose adrenergic fibers supplies virtually the entire brain, with the exception of a few very discrete regions (e.g., caudate nucleus). Noradrenaline released from this terminal plexus may influence any cellular elements with appropriate receptors. This influence would be accomplished through a neurohumoral mechanism rather than through classic synaptic specializations. Blood vessels and glial cells, both of which have adrenergic receptors, would be affected only by this type of innervation. Neurons, though possibly directly affected by this type of neurohumoral innervation, usually would be affected only indirectly by alteration in the extracellular fluid composition. Superimposed on this diffuse, rather slowly acting neurohumoral system are specific brain regions or groups of neurons that receive discrete and specific innervation via transmitter release at synaptic specializations. Examples of both types of adrenergic innervation [33] are shown in figures 1 and 2.

Physiologic Evidence for Central Adrenergic Regulation of Capillary Permeability

The cerebral microvasculature is the most extensively studied nonneuronal component of the brain that appears to be innervated by the central adrenergic system. In addition to anatomical evidence for innervation at the light and electron microscopic levels, the presence of adrenergic receptors on isolated cerebral capillaries has been demonstrated and characterized [6]. The purpose of this innervation appears to be regulation of capillary permeability.

We know that many compounds do not move freely across the cerebral capillaries, generally referred to as the blood-brain barrier. Originally, we

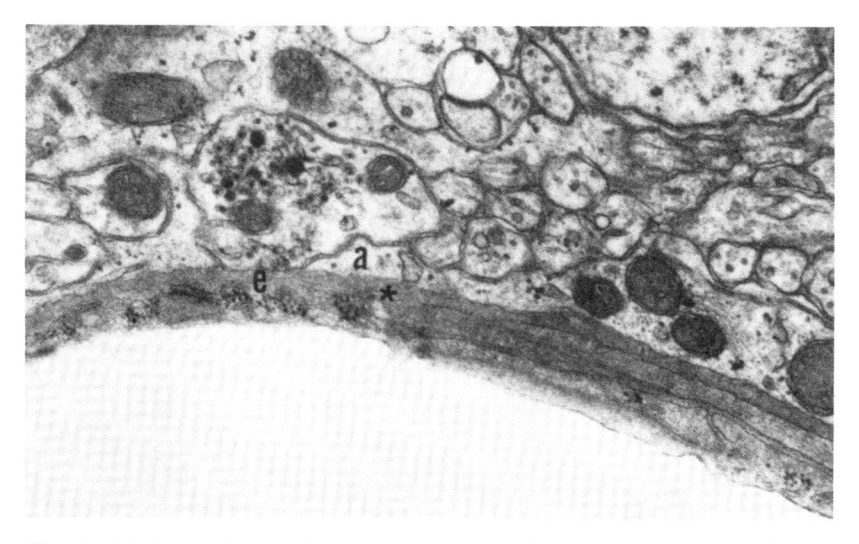

Fig. 1. Adrenergic innervation of a cerebral capillary. A dense-core vesicle-containing varicosity lying on the basal lamina of a capillary endothelial cell (e) in the paraventricular nucleus. The basal lamina splits to surround part of a pericyte or smooth muscle cell at the asterisk (*). The varicosity is partly surrounded by astrocytic processes (a). Ganglionectomized, 5-OHDA pretreated rat [5].
(Reprinted by permission from L.W. Swanson et al.: "Ultrastructural evidence for central monoaminergic innervation of blood vessels of paraventricular nucleus of the hypothalamus," *Brain Research*, Vol. 136, pp. 166–173. Copyright 1977, Elsevier/North Holland, Amsterdam.)

thought this barrier only affected the movement of complex compounds in a nonvariable either/or manner. However, we now know that this selective permeability extends to a wide variety of substances, including simple compounds such as water and short chain aliphatic alcohols [7].

The implications of neurogenic control of capillary permeability are numerous. It means that the brain may have a way of controlling its own internal composition and that malfunctions in these control mechanisms could indirectly affect normal functioning of the nervous system.

A variety of experiments indicate that neurogenic regulation of cerebral capillary permeability to water indeed occurs. Two independent methods have been used to evaluate the changes in capillary permeability to water. One method, which was developed in the Washington University School of Medicine [8], uses a single radioactive tracer, ^{15}O-labeled water. This method permits the simultaneous in vivo measurement of cerebral blood flow (CBF) and extraction fraction (E) of the diffusible tracer employed during a single capillary transit through the brain. An index of the capillary permeability of the tracer (PS) can be calculated from the values of E and CBF using the rela-

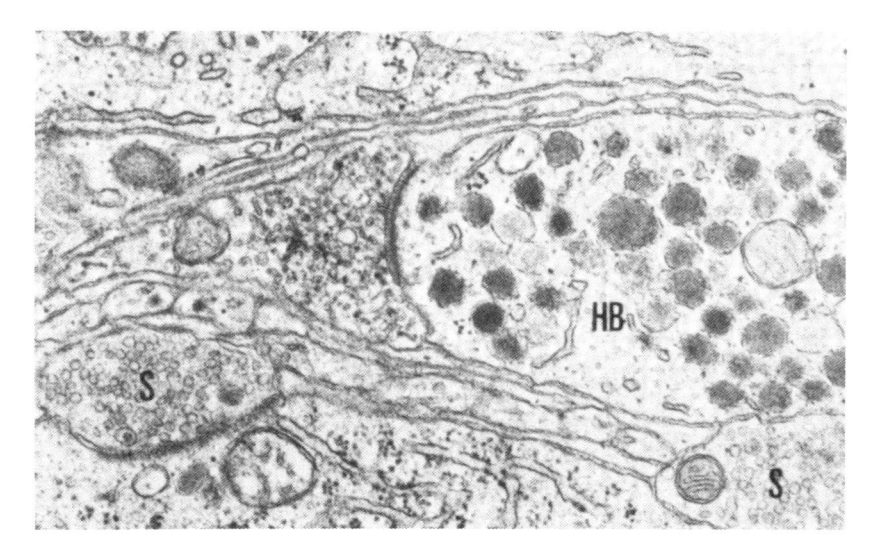

Fig. 2. Adrenergic innervation of a central neuron. An axoaxonic synapse(s) between a microgranular vesicle-containing varicosity and a neurosecretory granule-filled swelling (Herring body, HB) associated with a magnocellular neurosecretory neuron in the paraventricular nucleus [33].
(Reprinted by permission from L. W. Swanson et al.: "Further studies on the fine structure of the adrenergic innervation of the hypothalamus," *Brain Research,* Vol. 151, pp. 165–174. Copyright 1978, Elsevier/North Holland, Amsterdam.)

tionship ln $(I-E) = \frac{-PS}{CBF}$ derived by *Renkin* [9] and *Crone* [10]. The tracer must be produced at the time of the experiment because it has a short half-life (2 min) and requires the use of a cyclotron. Experiments using this methodology showed that, in the rhesus monkey, stimulation of the locus ceruleus resulted in a rapid increase in capillary permeability to water. This increase occurred when the central adrenergic cell bodies were stimulated either electrically [11] or chemically by microinjection of the cholinergic agonist, carbamylcholine [12]. Changes in blood flow could also be measured during stimulation. However, the magnitude and direction of the changes depend on the baseline flow at the beginning of the experiment. Capillary permeability to water could also be altered by intracerebroventricular injection of the alpha adrenergic blocking agent, phentolamine [12]. Furthermore, increases in permeability caused by prior stimulation of the locus ceruleus could be reversed by intraventricular administration of this antagonist [13] (fig. 3). In all cases,

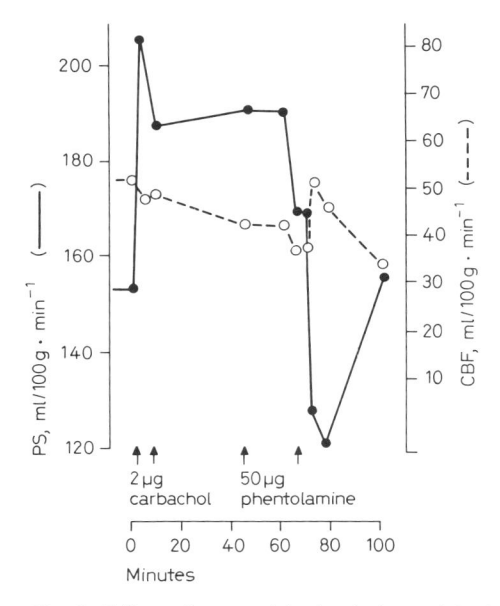

Fig. 3. Effect of sequential stimulations of the locus ceruleus by microinjections of carbamylcholine (2 μg in 1 μl) followed by blockade and reversal of the effect on capillary permeability (PS) with intraventricular administration of the alpha-adrenergic antagonist phentolamine (50 μg) in a bilaterally superiocervical ganglionectomized monkey. These pharmacologic manipulations did not result in significant alterations in cerebral blood flow (CBF) [13].
(Reprinted by permission from E. Usdin (ed.): *Catecholamines: Basic and Clinical Frontiers*, Vol. 1, pp. 450–452. Copyright 1978, Pergamon Press, Ltd., New York.)

changes in either capillary permeability or CBF were rapidly reversible and could not be explained by alterations in peripheral autonomic tone or by changes in blood gas concentrations. These experiments provide strong evidence that, in addition to altering the excitability of other neurons, the central adrenergic system also influences the nonneuronal elements of the brain.

Possible Physiologic Role of Neurogenic Regulation of CBF and Vascular Permeability

We have shown that both cerebral blood flow and capillary permeability to water can be affected by stimulation of the central adrenergic cell bodies. Furthermore, an effect in the opposite direction can be elicited by the administration of the alpha-adrenergic blocking agent, phentolamine. A functional hypothesis is evolving as to the possible necessity for such neurogenic mechanisms. So that the brain may function properly, a number of factors must be regulated within narrow limits. Mechanisms must be available to ensure cerebral blood flow regulation and constant brain volume (i.e., brain water content to prevent cerebral edema) in the face of changes in both perfusion pressure and serum osmolarity. Flow can be regulated by alterations in vascular resistance. However, changes in vascular resistance (at constant perfusion pressure) will result in changes in capillary pressure. This would lead to a net flux of water either into or out of the brain, with resulting alterations in brain volume or pressure. Similarly, changes in serum osmolarity as a result of water load or water deprivation would result in net fluxes of water into or out of the brain. A mechanism capable of regulating capillary permeability to water (i.e., PS) could prevent net movement of fluid in these circumstances.

Both effects described above occur in the monkey. An immediate increase in PS for water was observed in response to acute intracarotid injections of hyperosmolar solutions of either mannitol or urea [11, 14]. Given the initial limited permeability of water at equilibrium, this effect temporarily prevents water from leaving the brain. More recent experiments show the reverse is also true. An acute hypotonic injection into the carotid artery results in an immediate decrease in water permeability, again temporarily preventing a net water flux. A similar phenomenon is demonstrated with changes in pressure. In norcapnic or hypercapnic animals, a sudden increase in arterial pressure (via angiotensin or metaraminol infusion) results in a decrease of capillary PS for water [15]. Both changes tend to prevent a net flux of water. An additional experiment has been carried out which has relevance to possible functional mechanisms. Injecting antidiuretic hormone (ADH) into the lateral ventricles, investigators found an immediate, but reversible, increase in capillary permeability to water (i.e., a response similar to that observed with a hypertonic solution) [16].

Whether these effects are normally mediated through the central adrenergic system has not been established. However, anatomical pathways from the paraventricular nucleus to the CSF and adrenergic neurons of the brain stem have been observed [17, 18]. These pathways present a possible means for mediating the observed responses to changes in blood osmolarity via the central adrenergic system. Similarly, the anatomical connections between baroreceptor vagal afferents to the adrenergic neurons in the dorsal vagal complex are well established at the light microscopic level [19] and may provide a pathway for the observed alterations in capillary permeability in response to changes in blood pressure. In a recent study, acute increases in blood volume resulted in the decreased firing rate of locus ceruleus neurons via input from the vagus nerve [20]. Such an effect results in decreased capillary permeability, and prevents fluid fluxes into the brain which might otherwise result during hypervolemic states. Thus, the proposed regulation of CBF and vascular permeability by the central adrenergic system can be viewed as a mechanism by which the brain may maintain fluid homeostasis.

Effects of Tricyclic Antidepressants on Cerebral Vascular Permeability

The relationship between the central adrenergic system and the cerebral microvasculature is based on the evidence presented above. In this model, the biochemically and anatomically defined neuronal system effects on the end organ, within the brain, could be quantified readily in vivo. This model represents one of the few examples in which a neuron of central origin terminates on an end organ (i.e., the cerebral capillary), instead of on another neuron.

Tricyclic antidepressants (TCAs) are presumed to affect the adrenergic system centrally. Therefore, a series of studies testing this model, and investigating in rats the regulation of cerebral capillary permeability by the central adrenergic system, was carried out using tricyclic antidepressants.

We could not use the single tracer $H_2^{15}O$ technique for these experiments. This method, while useful in monkey experiments, is not applicable in smaller animals. Therefore, a different technique was used. This method consists of the relative extraction of a freely diffusible tracer (^{14}C-butanol) and a diffusion-limited test tracer (^3H-water or ^3H-ethanol) to determine the extraction fraction (E_w or E_e, respectively) of the test tracer. The method is a modification of the

Oldendorf technique [21]. When the blood flow is constant, E_w or E_e becomes an index of permeability [see 22–24 for details of the methodology].

Under control conditions, E_w equals $0.70 + 0.01$ [22, 23]. The small standard error of the mean reflects the reproducibility of this measure. It is especially meaningful considering these studies were carried out over an 18-month period. An E_w of 0.70 means that in one circulatory transit time, only 70% of the tracer entering the cerebral vascular compartment equilibrates with the central parenchymal compartment. This finding agrees with previous data showing that water is diffusion limited across the cerebral capillary [7, 8].

Based on the central adrenergic vasoregulatory hypothesis, we predicted that tricyclic antidepressants, acting as indirect adrenergic agonists, would cause an increase in E_w and E_e. We studied the tricyclic amitriptyline (AMI) most extensively. Acute intraperitoneal administration of AMI caused a rapid increase in both E_w (fig. 4) and E_e (fig. 5). The effect was reversible, dose-

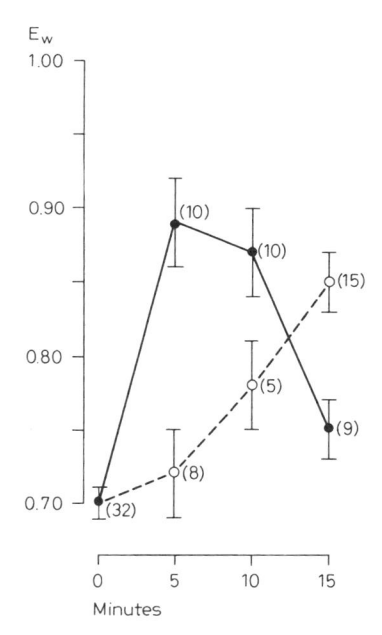

Fig. 4. Total forebrain E_w as a function of time and dose. ● = 125 μmol/kg dose. E_w was different from untreated controls (0 time point) at 5 and 10 min ($p < 0.001$) and at 15 min ($p < 0.05$). ○ = 62.5 μmol/kg. E_w was different from controls at 10 and 15 min ($p < 0.001$). Numbers in parentheses, number of animals [23].
(Reprinted by permission from S. Preskorn et al.: "The effects of dibenzazepines on cerebral capillary permeability in the rats in vivo," *The Journal of Pharmacology and Experimental Therapeutics,* Vol. 213, pp. 313–320, 1980. Copyright American Society for Pharmacology and Experimental Therapeutics.)

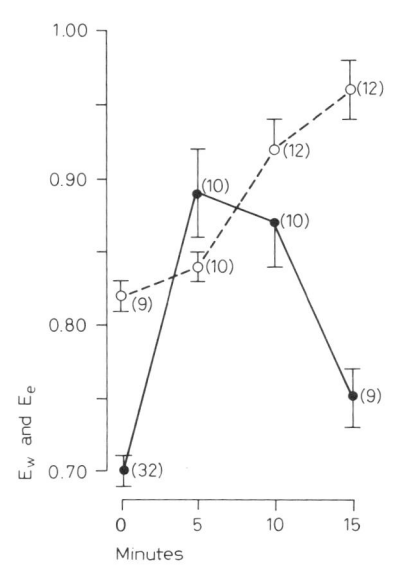

Fig. 5. Comparison of time-response curves for E_w (●) and E_e (○) for total forebrain after 125 μmol/kg of AMI. Numbers in parentheses, number of animals [23]. (Reprinted by permission from S. Preskorn et al.: "The effects of dibenzazepines on cerebral capillary permeability in the rats in vivo," *The Journal of Pharmacology and Experimental Therapeutics,* Vol. 213, pp. 313–320, 1980. Copyright American Society for Pharmacology and Experimental Therapeutics.)

dependent, and occurred uniformly through all brain regions studied (including rostral telencephalon, caudal telencephalon, diencephalon, brain stem, and cerebellum).

These findings have several important implications. The global nature and rapidity of the effect suggests that the drug exerts its effect via a mechanism common to all regions studied and that the drug affects the cerebral capillary membrane, either directly or indirectly, via a rapidly acting mechanism. The rapidity of the response is inconsistent with a mechanism requiring structural alteration of the membrane by protein synthesis. Furthermore, the response is transient, demonstrating that it reflects a functional alteration rather than a destruction of membrane integrity. These findings are consistent with the drug exerting this effect via a central neural system whose function is regulation of cerebral capillary permeability.

Other mechanisms of action, however, are also possible. The tricyclic antidepressants are complex pharmacologic agents with a wide variety of actions. Their blockade of catecholamine reuptake is well known [25]. They also block reuptake of serotonin [26]. In addition, they have binding affinity for both muscarinic and catecholaminergic receptors [27, 28], and have potent anticholinergic effects. Moreover, tricyclic antidepressants possess important direct effects on membrane properties [29]. They are potent local anesthetics, they inhibit the hypoosmotic hemolysis of red blood cells, and they can lower the surface tension of solutions.

The anticholinergic actions of the TCAs probably are not important in altering central permeability, since atropine was shown not to affect E_w. Destruction of the serotonergic system with the neurotoxin p-chloramphetamine did not alter the effect of AMI on E_w, indicating that the serotonin system is not involved in this effect. The idea is more likely that the central adrenergic system mediates the AMI-induced increase in E_w. The effect is blocked by pretreatment with phenoxybenzamine, an alpha-adrenergic antagonist, and by intraventricular administration of 6-hydroxydopamine, a selective catecholaminergic neurotoxin. The phenoxybenzamine blockade occurs in a dose-dependent manner. Using phenoxybenzamine pretreatment, we attenuated the increase in E_w induced by AMI (125 μmol/kg) by 70%. Phenoxybenzamine, however, did not alter E_w in the absence of AMI. Since tricyclic antidepressants act as indirect adrenergic agonists by blocking the reuptake of norepinephrine, they are dependent on an intact, functioning adrenergic fiber. Based on the concept that AMI increases E_w via this adrenergic mechanism, we correctly predicted that the AMI-induced increase would be blocked by ablation of the central adrenergic system by 6-hydroxydopamine. Figure 6 schematically summarizes the pharmacologic evidence supporting the central adrenergic mediation TCA-induced alterations in capillary permeability. Another interesting aspect of AMI-induced increase in E_w is the finding of an inverted U-shaped relationship between tricyclic (amitriptyline + nortriptyline) concentration in the brain and the alteration in E_w (fig. 7). This effect appears to occur only within a certain concentration range, suggesting that at higher concentrations the drug blocks its initial action. At low concentrations, these drugs act as adrenergic agonists by blocking norepinephrine reuptake. At higher concentrations, they are potent local anesthetics and their membrane-stabilizing properties predominate [29]. It is not known whether a similar mechanism underlies the concentration-effect relationship reported here. However, these results are the first in vivo examples of an inverted U-shaped relationship between concentration and response in the central nervous system. This resembles the reported window effect seen in patients treated with nortriptyline, the major metabolite of amitriptyline.

Although AMI was the prototype, all TCAs were tested as to their ability to induce an increase in cerebral capillary permeability to water. Although all

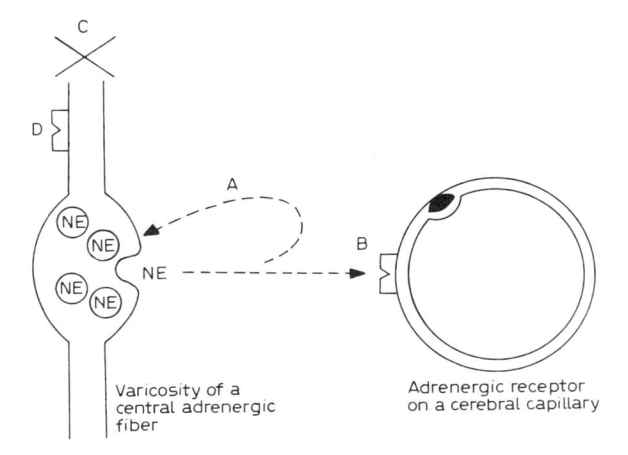

Fig. 6. Schematic diagram representing proposed sites of drug actions [34]. A = Primary effects of TCAs blockade of NE reuptake into presynaptic varicosity, thereby increasing NE concentration at capillary receptor. B = Pretreatment with phenoxybenzamine (an alpha-adrenergic receptor blocker) blocks the effect of TCAs at capillary receptor to increase cerebral capillary permeability. C = Ablation of the central adrenergic system via 6-hydroxydopamine pretreatment blocks the tricyclic antidepressant-induced increase in cerebral capillary permeability. D = Chronic TCA administration enhances the alteration in cerebral capillary permeability, possibly by action on presynaptic receptors.
(Reprinted by permission from S.H. Preskorn and B.K. Hartman: "Tricyclic antidepressants: New sites of action," *Behavioral Medicine*, Vol. 6, No. 11, pp. 30–33, 1979.)

tricyclic antidepressants produced this change, marked differences in potency were observed. Table I shows the results of this experiment expressed as change in the permeability coefficient compared with control. Doxepin produced the greatest alteration in permeability (240% of control) and protriptyline the least (130% of control). The rank order of TCAs based on the effect of the drugs on E_w, 5 min after a 125 μmol/kg dose i.p., is as follows: doxepin > AMI > imipramine > NOR > desmethylimipramine > protriptyline. This rank order correlates well ($r = 0.93$) with the alpha-adrenergic receptor binding affinities of these compounds [28]. Thus, the relative potency results are also compatible with an action involving the central adrenergic system.

Since these drugs are used extensively in clinical practice, the question arises whether this effect may occur in man. Three observations support this possibility. First, the effect occurs in rats after acute treatment at tricyclic plasma concentrations between 500 and 1,000 ng/ml. These levels are higher than the AMI therapeutic range for man (160–240 ng/ml) [30, 31]. However,

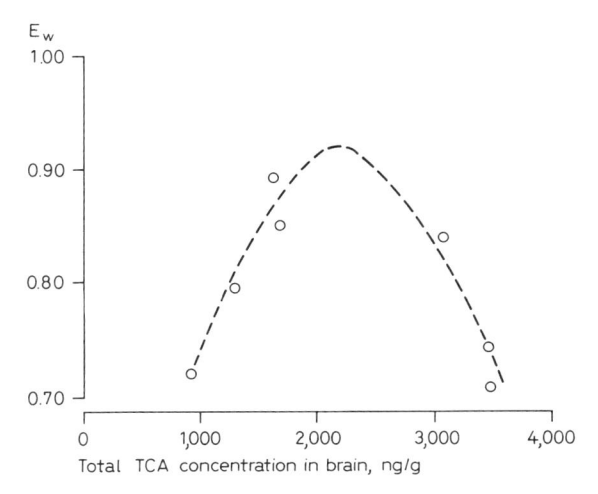

Fig. 7. Total forebrain E_w as a function of total tricyclic (AMI + NOR) concentration in brain (ng/g wet weight tissue). A curvilinear relationship also held when plotted against AMI or NOR concentrations separately. E_w returned to near baseline values at 15 min with the 125 μmol/kg dose ($E_w = 0.71$) and at 30 min with the 62.5 μmol/kg dose ($E_w = 0.74$). At these times, the brain concentrations were almost identical: ($\bar{X}$) 3,496 and 3,476 ng/g, respectively. Each point represents results from 5 to 15 animals. TCA = Tricyclic antidepressants [23].
(Reprinted by permission from S. Preskorn et al.: "The effects of dibenzazepines on cerebral capillary permeability in the rats in vivo," *The Journal of Pharmacology and Experimental Therapeutics*, Vol. 213, pp. 313–320, 1980. Copyright American Society for Pharmacology and Experimental Therapeutics.)

Table 1. Calculated changes in the total forebrain capillary permeability coefficient (P_w) of water as a function of drug treatment (125 μmol/kg) [23]

Group	n	$\dfrac{(P_w) \text{ treatment}}{(P_w) \text{ control}}$, %
Controls	32	100
Doxepin	14	240
Amitriptyline	10	184
Imipramine	12	173
Nortriptyline	10	159
Desmethylimipramine	12	146
Protriptyline	12	130

(Reprinted by permission from S. Preskorn et al.: "The effects of dibenzazepines on cerebral capillary permeability in the rats in vivo," *The Journal of Pharmacology and Experimental Therapeutics*, Vol. 213, pp. 313–320, 1980. Copyright American Society for Pharmacology and Experimental Therapeutics.)

the therapeutic range is determined in postdistribution, steady state conditions, while the plasma levels in these animals are predistribution and thus will overshoot the therapeutic range. Second, the effect occurs in monkeys at tricyclic plasma concentrations ranging from 100 to 200 ng/ml. Finally, this vascular effect is enhanced by chronic treatment [32]. In this study, rats were treated with the 62.5 μmol/kg i.p. dose of AMI twice daily for 2 weeks without fatality. Half the animals received a morning dose 5 min before measurement of E_w; the other half received no morning dose, E_w being measured 12 h after drug administration. E_w in the former group was 0.98 ± 0.04, which is higher than the E_w seen with acute treatment at double the dose (125 μmol/kg). E_w in the latter group was 0.80 ± 0.02, which represents a sustained increase in the permeability of water across the cerebral capillary throughout the dosing interval and 12 h after drug administration. The tricyclic plasma concentration in these animals was 70 ± 13 ng/ml. Thus, the effect was enhanced by chronic treatment producing steady state drug conditions resembling clinical pharmacotherapy. Based on these observations, it seems likely that AMI and the other tricyclic antidepressants produce this alteration in blood-brain barrier permeability in patients being treated for depression.

This report reviews the evidence that tricyclic antidepressants have potent effects on the selective permeability of cerebral capillaries and thus emphasizes that psychoactive drugs may have important central effects on nonneuronal tissue components. Moreover, the biologic importance of these results should be underscored. If these drugs can affect the permeability coefficients of both polar and lipid-soluble substances, other more complex substances such as glucose, amino acids, or other drugs may also become more permeable when the organism is treated with TCAs. Changes in the cerebral capillary permeability of such substances would be expected to have profound effects on brain fluid dynamics, metabolism, and possibly other aspects of cerebral function.

Conclusion

The central adrenergic system has been shown to have many anatomical and physiologic similarities to the peripheral sympathetic nervous system. The widespread distribution of its efferent terminal plexuses and the structures they innervate as well as its numerous afferent connections indicate that this system plays a role in the regulation of the internal environment of the brain in response to external events. We have emphasized effects on nonneuronal elements which occur through neurohumoral mechanisms, but evidence is equally strong supporting direct local synaptic effects on individual neurons. We hypothesized that both effects have the same overall function; that is, to maintain cerebral homeostasis in the broadest possible sense. For example, in a fluid deprivation situation, alterations occur in cerebral capillary permeability to prevent fluid loss from the brain, antidiuretic hormone release is stimulated to prevent further loss of fluid, and on a higher cortical level one also experiences the subjective cognitive feeling of thirst. Anatomical pathways are known by which the central adrenergic system could initiate and mediate all three of these specific functions. The net result is, first, to maintain homeostasis temporarily with the materials at hand and, second, to stimulate appropriate fluid searching behavior to solve the problem.

We assume that many of the recently described divergent neuronal systems (containing vasopressin, oxytocin, enkephalin, endorphin and other peptides) are also involved in intra-axial autonomic regulatory functions of this type. It is not inconceivable that the cognitive interpretation by the patient of the effects of a disregulation of these basic central autonomic mechanisms is what we call depression and which takes the clinical form of sleep and appetite disturbances, difficulty in concentration, low interest and motivation, and general malaise. The multiple divergent neuronal systems that seem to mediate these central homeostatic functions do not act independently, but clearly work in concert by continuous interactions with each other. It seems, therefore, that debate and investigation aimed at determining which single neuron system or single transmitter is specially responsible for depression is unlikely to be productive.

Similarly, as can be seen from the perhaps unexpected but marked influence of TCAs on cerebral capillary permeability, one should be cautious in oversimplifying the mechanism of action of these complex drugs. We are likely just starting to scratch the surface of completely understanding all that occurs in the nervous system of patients under treatment with psychotherapeutic agents.

Acknowledgments

This work was supported in part by the following grants from the National Institutes of Health: NS-12311, NS-13672, NS-06833, NS-10943, NS-13267, HL-13851 and Research Scientist Development Award MH-70451 (Dr. *Boyd K. Hartman*).

References

1 Hartman, B.K.; Udenfriend, S.: The application of immunological techniques to the study of enzymes regulating catecholamine synthesis and degradation. Pharmac. Rev. *24:* 311 (1972).
2 Dahlström, A.; Fuxe, K.: Evidence for the existence of monoamine-containing neurons in the central nervous system. I. Demonstration of monoamines in the cell bodies of brain stem neurons. Acta physicol. scand. *62:* suppl. 232, pp. 1–55 (1964).
3 Hartman, B.K.; Zide, D.; Udenfriend, S.: The use of dopamine-β-hydroxylase as a marker for the central noradrenergic nervous system in the rat brain. Proc. natn. Acad. Sci. USA *69:* 2722 (1972).
4 Hartman, B.K.; The innervation of cerebral blood vessels by central noradrenergic neurons; in Frontiers in catecholamine research, pp. 91–96 (Pergamon Press, Oxford 1973).
5 Swanson, L.W.; Connelly, M.A.; Hartman, B.K.: Ultrastructural evidence for central monoaminergic innervation of blood vessels of paraventricular nucleus of the hypothalamus. Brain Res. *136:* 166–173 (1977).
6 Herbst, T.J.; Raichle, M.E.; Ferrendelli, J.A.: β-Adrenergic regulation of adenosine 3', 5'-monophosphate concentration in brain microvessels. Science N.Y. *204:* 330–332 (1979).
7 Raichle, M.E.; Eichling, J.O.; Straatmann, M.G.; Welch, M.J.; Larson, K.B.; Ter-Pogossian, M.M.: Blood-brain barrier permeability of ^{11}C-labeled alcohols and ^{15}O-labeled water. Am. J. Physiol. *230:* 543–552 (1976).
8 Eichling, J.O.; Raichle, M.E.; Grubb, R.L.; Ter-Pogossian, M.M.: Evidence of the limitations of water as a freely diffusible tracer in brain of the rhesus monkey. Circulation Res. *35:* 358–364 (1974).
9 Renkin, E.M.: Transport of potassium-42 from blood to tissue in isolated mammalian skeletal muscles. Am. J. Physiol. *197:* 1205–1210 (1959).
10 Crone, C.: Permeability of capillaries in various organs as determined by use of the indicator diffusion method. Acta physiol. scand. *58:* 292–305 (1963).
11 Raichle, M.E.; Eichling, J.O; Grubb, R.L; Hartman, B.K.: Central noradrenergic regulation of brain microcirculation; in Hanna, Pappius, Feindel, Dynamics of brain edema, pp. 11–17 (Springer, Berlin 1976).
12 Raichle, M.E.; Hartman, B.K.; Eichling, J.O.; and Sharpe, L.G.: Central noradrenergic regulation of cerebral blood flow and vascular permeability. Proc. natn. Acad. Sci. USA *72:* 3726–3730 (1975).
13 Hartman, B.K.; Swanson, L.W.; Raichle, M.E.; Clark, H.B.; Preskorn, S.H.: Evidence for central adrenergic regulation of cerebral vascular permeability and blood flow; in Usdin, Catecholamines: basic and clinical frontiers, pp. 450–452 (Pergamon Press, Oxford 1978).
14 Raichle, M.E.; Grubb, R.L., Jr.; Eichling, J.O.: Osmotically induced changes in brain water permeability. Fed. Proc. *36:* 470 (1977).
15 Raichle, M.E.; Grubb, R.L., Jr.: Acute arterial hypertension and brain water permeability. Fed. Proc. *37:* 242 (1978).

16 Raichle, M.E.; Grubb, R.L., Jr.: Regulation of brain water permeability by centrally-released vasopressin. Brain Res. *143:* 191–194 (1978).

17 Swanson, L.W.: Immunohistochemical evidence for a neurophysin-containing autonomic pathway arising in the paraventricular nucleus of the hypothalamus. Brain Res. *128:* 346–353 (1977).

18 Swanson, L.W.; Hartman, B.K.: Biochemical specificity in central pathways related to peripheral and intracerebral homeostatic functions. Neurosci. Lett. *16:* 55–60 (1980).

19 Swanson, L.W.; Hartman, B.K.: The central adrenergic system. An immunofluorescence study of the location of cell bodies and their efferent connections in the rat utilizing dopamine-β-hydroxylase as a marker. J. comp. Neurol. *163:* 467–505 (1975).

20 Svensson, T.H.; Thoren, P.: Brain noradrenergic neurons in the locus coeruleus: inhibition by blood volume load through vagal afferents. Brain Res. *172:* 174–178 (1979).

21 Oldendorf, W.: Measurement of brain uptake of radio-labeled substances using a tritiated water internal standard. Brain Res. *24:* 372–376 (1970).

22 Preskorn, S.; Hartman, B.K.: The effect of tricyclic antidepressants on cerebral fluid dynamics. Biol. Psychiat. *14:* 235–250 (1979).

23 Preskorn, S.; Hartman, B.K.; Raichle, M.; Clark, H.B.: The effects of dibenzazepines on cerebral capillary permeability in the rats in vivo. J. Pharmac. exp. Ther. *213:* 313–320 (1980).

24 Preskorn, S.; Hartman, B.K.; Raichle, M.; Clark, H.B.: Amitriptyline induced alterations in cerebral capillary permeability. Neurosci. Abstr. *4:* 500 (1978).

25 Ross, S.; Renyi, A.: Inhibition of the uptake of tritiated catecholamines by antidepressants and related agents. Eur. J. Pharmacol. *2:* 181–186 (1967).

26 Alpers, H.; Hinwich, H.: An in vitro study of the effects of tricyclic antidepressant drugs on the accumulation of ^{14}C-serotonin by rabbit brain. Biol. Psychiat. *1:* 81–85 (1969).

27 Snyder, S.; Yamamura, H.: Antidepressants and the muscarinic acetylcholine receptor. Archs. gen. Psychiat. *34:* 236–239 (1977).

28 U'Prichard, D.; Greenberg, D.; Sheehan, P., et al.: Tricyclic antidepressants: therapeutic properties and affinity for alpha-noradrenergic receptor binding sites in the brain. Science, N.Y. *199:* 197–198 (1977).

29 Elonen, E.: Correlation of the cardiotoxicity of the tricyclic antidepressants to their membrane effects. Med. Biol. *52:* 415–423 (1974).

30 Ziegler, V.; Co, B.; Taylor, J.; Clayton, P.; Biggs, J.: Amitriptyline plasma levels and therapeutic response. Clin. Pharmacol. Ther. *19:* 795–801 (1976).

31 Preskorn, S.; Biggs, J.: Use of tricyclic antidepressant blood levels. New Engl. J. Med. *298:* 166 (1978).

32 Preskorn, S.; Hartman, B.; Clark, H.: Long-term antidepressant treatment: effect on cerebral capillary permeability. Psychopharmacology (in press, 1980).

33 Swanson, L.W.; Connelly, M.A.; Hartman, B.K.: Further studies on the fine structure of the adrenergic innervation of the hypothalamus. Brain Res. *151:* 165–174 (1978).

34 Preskorn, S.H.; Hartman, B.K.: Tricyclic antidepressants: new sites of action. Behav. Med. 6: 30–33 (1979).

Discussion

Mendels: How do your studies apply to the antidepressant effects of the tricyclic drugs?

Hartman: The relationship between tricyclic effects on capillary permeability and the antidepressant effects of these drugs is not known. We look at the vasoregulatory effects as an in vivo model system by which we can measure a specific central neurogenic response to these drugs. Nevertheless, if our concept of depression as a dysregulation of general central homeostatic mechanisms is correct, a number of important implications follow. First, many different neuronal systems and transmitters may be involved in depression and to attempt defining all depressions as a defect in any one or even two particular transmitters is probably a great oversimplification. Second, it is probably a mistake at this point to invoke one particular pharmacologic test as indicative of whether a given antidepressant affects a particular neuron system. For example, doxepin and amitriptyline are not potent with respect to blocking norepinephrine reuptake as measured in in vitro systems. Yet they are the most potent TCAs as to their binding affinity for the alpha-noradrenergic receptor, and they have the greatest effect on capillary permeability, which is apparently mediated through the central noradrenergic system. Furthermore, both drugs are excellent antidepressants; but so are TCAs which have lower alpha-noradrenergic receptor affinity and capillary permeability effects. The point is that given the existence of multiple types of receptors at multiple physiologic sites on neurons and postsynaptic cells, it is not possible to deduce on the basis of any single test what the net resultant effect will be in vivo on the central noradrenergic system (or any other system).

Hawkins: When you refer to sympathetic, are you thinking of sympathetic or autonomic functions in general?

Hartman: I think the central adrenergic system is analogous to the peripheral sympathetic system in terms of the functions it mediates. I believe it plays a major role in central autonomic regulation. In the past, it has generally been assumed that factors such as cerebral blood flow and brain water content were maintained without the need for neurogenic mechanisms as supplied by the sympathetic system in the periphery. For example, it was assumed that if excess fluid entered the brain because of an increase in blood pressure, the resultant increased intracranial pressure would cause additional CSF adsorption into the blood on the venous side, thereby reducing cerebral pressure back to normal. The advantage of a neurogenic mechanism over such autoregulatory mechanisms is that potential problems can be anticipated and action taken to prevent a problem from developing rather than responding after the fact. Thus, with a neurogenic mechanism, if the blood pressure increases, the central adrenergic system is made aware of this fact via vagal sensory afferents from baroreceptors, and adrenergic efferents to the blood vessels can reduce capillary permeability accordingly. This would prevent fluid from entering the brain in the first place and negate the need for the brain to withstand the increase in pressure necessary to activate an autoregulatory mechanism.

Hawkins: Some of the anatomical areas you mentioned, such as the locus ceruleus, are important in sleep and cyclic rhythms. There is increasing evidence that these areas also are in some way connected with depression. Have you studied the effect, over time, on circadian rhythm in your system?

Hartman: No. However, other investigators have looked at the firing of the locus ceruleus during REM sleep. There is no question that the central adrenergic system is altered. However, whether this has anything to do with depression or with antidepressant drugs has yet to be determined.

Maas: Do cerebral permeability changes ever occur solely as a function of cerebral blood flow? For example, if one alters CBF by altering pCO_2, is permeability altered?

Hartman: We cannot test this directly in rats. However, in the monkey, where we use a method that distinguishes between permeability and flow, we haven't observed altered permeability in response to changes in cerebral blood flow.

Lipton: Have you studied the permeability of any nutrients?

Hartman: We don't have any data on glucose or the amino acids, because the model for understanding transport of these compounds is much more complex. Unlike water, these other substances are influenced by active transport, facilitated transport, and other factors which are less easily measured. However, I guess that if a simple substance like water is affected, the same membrane effects would alter the transport of more complex compounds as well.

Doxepin: Recent Pharmacologic and Clinical Studies

Steven K. Secunda

Clinical Research Branch, National Institute of Mental Health, Bethesda, Maryland

This paper presents recent pharmacologic and clinical information concerning the tricyclic antidepressant (TCA), doxepin. The primary emphasis is on reviewing clinical studies (fig. 1) to define a unique clinical spectrum for doxepin in the treatment of the depressive disorders. Pharmacodynamic studies are reviewed briefly, with appropriate references cited for the reader interested in examining these aspects in greater detail.

Drug Studies

Many studies have compared doxepin with other available tricyclic antidepressants or placebo to determine doxepin's efficacy.

In 1974, *Morris and Beck* [14] published a review of controlled double-blind studies on the efficacy of antidepressant drugs conducted from 1958 to 1972. At that time, three studies on the treatment of depression showed no difference in efficacy between doxepin and imipramine. Of eight reports comparing doxepin with amitriptyline, three found doxepin significantly more effective than amitriptyline, one found it less effective, and four found no differences between the two drugs. Therefore, doxepin appeared as effective an antidepressant as the other tricyclic drugs.

However, I believe that many of those clinicians who consider doxepin less effective than either imipramine or amitriptyline rarely prescribe dosages exceeding 75–100 mg/day. This is at least 50 mg below the recommended dose range of 150–300 mg/day. Underdosing is the chief reason for therapeutic drug failure.

Over the years, studies have shown that all TCAs, including doxepin, are

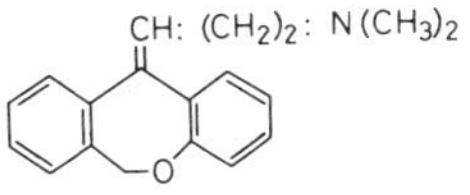

Fig. 1. Structures of doxepin, amitriptyline and imipramine.
(Reprinted with permission from R.N. Pinder, et al.: "Doxepin: A review of the pharmacologic properties and therapeutic efficacy with particular reference to depression," *Drugs,* Vol. 13, pp. 161–218, 1977. Sydney, Australia and New York: Adis Press, Ltd.)

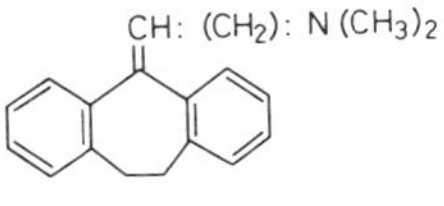

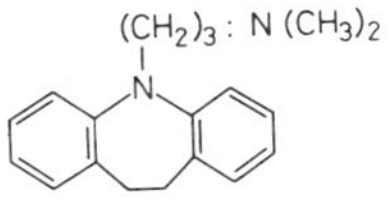

equally effective if given in adequate doses. Among these were the studies of *Grof* et al. [15] comparing doxepin with amitriptyline, using daily dosages of 150–350 mg for doxepin and 100–200 mg for amitriptyline. *Castrogiovanni* et al. [16] compared doxepin with imipramine, using a mean daily dosage of 222 mg of doxepin, and a mean dosage of 200 mg of imipramine. They found no differences in overall efficacies, although imipramine appeared to act more rapidly.

More recently, *Mendels* et al., [17] compared the efficacy and safety of doxepin and imipramine. They used a randomized double-blind design in outpatients with psychoneurosis, symptoms of anxiety, depression, and sleep disturbances. The dosage range was 50–250 mg/day of doxepin and 50–200 mg/day for imipramine. These authors found that patients exhibited similar improvement of symptoms with doxepin and imipramine. However, doxepin seemed to produce improved quality of sleep (relative to imipramine) by the 1st week of therapy. Based on previous studies, clinicians considered imipramine the drug of choice for retarded depression, while doxepin was favored for patients with depression accompanied by symptoms of anxiety. In this study, however, it was demonstrated (using the Hamilton Depression Scale Retardation Factor, the Hamilton Depression Scale Somatization/Anxiety Factor, and the Poms Tension/Anxiety Factor) that doxepin is as effective as if not more effective than imipramine for patients with severe depressive retardation. Interestingly, doxepin also is at least as effective as imipramine in relieving anxiety in its psychologic aspect (Poms Tension/Anxiety Factor), and when anxiety is combined with somatic symptoms of anxiety and depression (Hamilton Somatization/Anxiety Factor) in patients with severe psychopathology [17].

Pharmacology

While it is clear that doxepin is an effective antidepressant, the mechanism of action of doxepin is not fully understood. According to the biogenic amine hypothesis, depression results from a decrease in amine neurotransmitters at receptors sites [1]. The tricyclic antidepressants have been thought to exert their effects by inhibiting the amine reuptake pump in presynaptic nerve endings in the brain, thus making more amine available and reversing the deficiency of neurotransmitters at the synapse. Compared with other TCAs, doxepin is only a weak inhibitor of norepinephrine or serotonin uptake into the peripheral organs or brain [2, 3]. Initially, perhaps for this reason, doxepin was considered a weak antidepressant. Early studies, using inadequate dosages of doxepin, appeared to confirm this. With the introduction of newer drugs, such as iprindole and mianserin, which have antidepressant actions clinically but no effect on biogenic amine uptake, it became apparent that the latter property may be of no clinical importance in the treatment of depression. Thus, the finding that doxepin is not an active potent inhibitor of norepinephrine or serotonin uptake may not be relevant to its effectiveness as an antidepressant, and other mechanisms may be involved in its efficacy. Indeed, because it does not have an effect on the norepinephrine system, this may make doxepin a preferable drug for depressed patients with coexisting heart disease.

Frazer, in this symposium, suggests that tricyclic antidepressants act by decreasing beta-adrenergic binding sites in brain, even without affecting norepinephrine uptake or monoamine oxidase activity. They also may alter the sensitivity of receptors. It is possible, therefore, that drugs such as doxepin exert their antidepressant effects by decreasing adrenergic reactivity.

The site of action of tricyclic antidepressants may be on the postsynaptic membrane [4]. Doxepin potentiates the synaptic inhibitory effect of biogenic amines. Doxepin and imipramine are indistinguishable in their dose-dependent potentiation of the inhibitory effect of norepinephrine on electrically induced postsynaptic (ganglionic) potentials [5] (fig. 2).

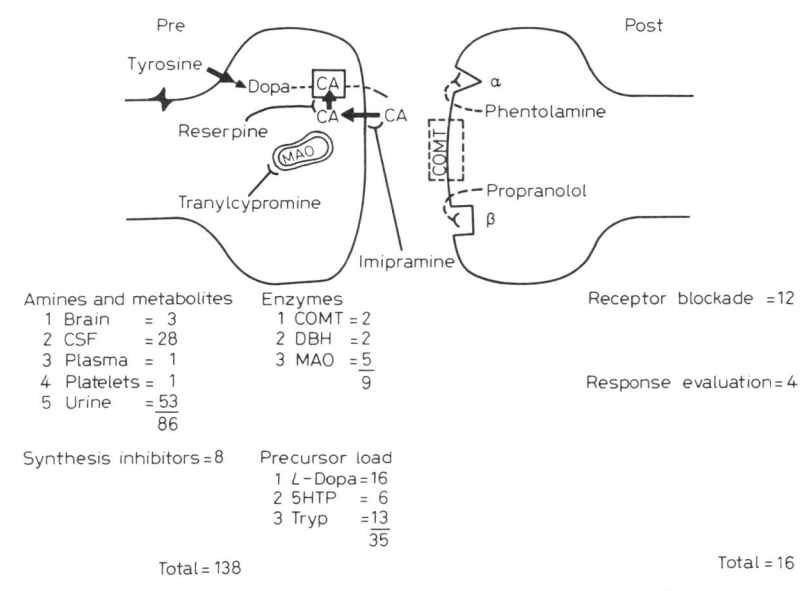

Doxepin: Recent Pharmacologic and Clinical Studies 133

Fig. 2. Schematic representation of a catecholaminergic neuron impinging on an effector cell. Sites of action of drugs which can modify such synaptic transmission are indicated. At the bottom of the figure is listed the number of original clinical investigations concerned with some aspects of DA, NE, or serotonin function in mania or depression [adapted from ref. 4].
(Reprinted by permission from Joseph Mendels, (ed.): *The Psychobiology of Depression,* Chapter 2, page 8, Figure 1. Copyright 1975, Spectrum Publications, Inc., New York.)

The enzyme adenylate cyclase is considered important in mediating the effects of hormones and neurotransmitters within the postsynaptic membrane. Doxepin inhibition of adenylate cyclase is as potent as amitriptyline inhibition and more potent than imipramine or desipramine inhibition [6].

Tricyclic antidepressants have an antihistamine property. Histamine may serve as a neurotransmitter and act by activation of H_1 and H_2 receptors. Doxepin has the greatest affinity for H_1 receptors of all the TCAs and ranks as the most potent antihistamine [7]. After doxepin, the order of potency is amitriptyline, imipramine, nortriptyline, protriptyline and desipramine. This correlates well with the drugs' sedative properties. Doxepin is more sedating than the other drugs mentioned. This characteristic may relate to the overall clinical effectiveness of doxepin in relieving target symptoms of depression. Further investigations may confirm this.

Doxepin, like other tricyclic antidepressants, has both peripheral and central anticholinergic activity [8]. In vitro studies, using models of central and peripheral muscarinic receptors (those with atropine-like activity), showed that doxepin is one-fourth as potent as amitriptyline at both receptors. Imipramine, which is equipotent at both central and peripheral muscarinic receptors, is more potent than doxepin in its ability to block muscarinic activity at the peripheral receptors as well as in its agonist characteristics. However, imipramine is less potent than doxepin at the central receptors [9]. The relatively low anticholinergic action of doxepin may be an important consideration in the treatment of depressed elderly patients for whom the discomfort of anticholinergic side effects may be accentuated (see below).

Doxepin is a derivative of dibenzoxepin and is structurally related to other tricyclic antidepressants such as amitriptyline and imipramine (fig. 1). Doxepin shares a similar profile of clinical action with amitriptyline in that it combines antidepressant activity with a sedative effect.

There is no agreement on the relationship between therapeutic response and TCA plasma levels. Therapeutic drug levels of TCAs must be achieved if the drugs are to be clinically effective. Underdosing appears to be a major cause of therapeutic failures. While there is some correlation between an oral dose of 150 mg or more of doxepin and therapeutic response, it was thought that plasma levels might correlate better with therapeutic response than does oral dosage. The results of plasma drug level studies, however, on the correlation of plasma TCA level and therapeutic response have been contradictory. One reason for this may be that blood collected via Vacutainer tubes shows lower plasma TCA level measurments than blood collected via glass heparinized syringes or Venoject tubes [10]. A chemical in the rubber stopper of the Vacutainer tube causes red blood cells to absorb increased levels of tricyclic drugs, thereby artificially lowering plasma TCA levels. This response is time-related.

Of the studies correlating plasma levels of doxepin and desmethyldoxepin to clinical response, *Kline* et al. [11] showed that the antidepressant efficacy of doxepin correlates significantly with plasma levels of desmethyldoxepin but not with doxepin itself. In a study of 50 elderly depressed patients (60 years old or older), *Friedel and Raskind* [12] found that plasma levels of doxepin plus desmethyldoxepin must exceed 110 ng/ml before most patients will show a therapeutic response. Seven patients who experienced little or no response had plasma levels averaging 60 ng/ml. The mean daily oral dose of doxepin was 104 mg for the nonresponders and 164 mg for the responders.

In another study, 17 of 21 patients with moderate to severe depression showed significant improvement with doxepin [13]. Most patients responded to a dosage range of doxepin between 2.1 and 3.9 mg/kg, with an average therapeutic daily dose of 196 mg, the majority of plasma levels ranging from 128 to 364 ng/ml. From this study, it appears that the plasma levels of doxepin, unlike other TCAs, are relatively predictable.

Cardiovascular Effects

Tricyclic antidepressants exert three separate pharmacologic actions on the heart: anticholinergic, adrenolytic and quinidine-like effects. The anticholinergic effects may include increased heart rate. The adrenolytic effects may include decreased heart rate, decreased cardiac output, and possibly hypotension. The quinidine-like effects may include decreased excitability, conduction velocity, and contraction of the heart. These actions are dose-related and have particular significance in the treatment of elderly depressed patients (see below).

Animal Studies
Slow intravenous injection of therapeutic doses of tricyclic antidepressants lowers blood pressure, increases heart rate, and frequently provokes severe arrhythmias in most animal species [18]. Studies in rabbits treated acutely in this manner with different TCAs showed a development of drug-induced cardiotoxicity. Drugs most potent in potentiating norepinephrine pressor responses, owing to inhibition of norepinephrine reuptake, were the most cardiotoxic. Therefore, doxepin, which is not a potent inhibitor of the amine pump, had the lowest cardiotoxicity [18]. When animals were treated with higher than therapeutic doses of the TCAs, however, all the drugs caused disturbances in membrane excitability and conduction, evidenced by decreased heart rate, partial or complete atrioventricular block, and QRS abnormalities such as right and left bundle branch blocks [11, 19, 20].

Clinical Studies
Inhibition of catecholamine reuptake by some tricyclic antidepressants results in blockade of the antihypertensive effects of guanethidine and enhancement of the pressor effects of sympathomimetic amines. Since doxepin has a poor inhibitory effect on the norepinephrine pump (compared with other TCAs), a daily dose of 200 mg or more is required before the drug antagonizes

guanethidine's antihypertensive effect in man [21, 22]. This correlates with clinical studies showing that daily doxepin doses of 200–300 mg were required before significant effects on biogenic amine metabolism appeared [21, 23].

While we do not have data on the incidence of cardiovascular disease in depressed patients, we do know that the reported incidence of depression in the elderly is increasing. Depressed elderly patients account for 25% of the total suicides in any given year. We also know that cardiovascular disease increases with age: 40 million Americans have some form of heart disease; 1 in 6 adults has hypertension [24]. Three-fourths of the persons dying from cardiovascular disease are over age 65. Diseases of the heart were the leading complaint of patients in this age group consulting physicians in 1977 [25]. Therefore, the prevalence of cardiovascular disease and hypertension in the age group 65 years and over suggests that these conditions should be considered in older depressed patients.

Interestingly, in a survey of 67,000 ECGs taken from presumably healthy air force personnel, 5.2/1,000 ECGs showed significant first-degree atrioventricular block [26]. Of subjects with cardiovascular disease, 10% have bundle branch block. Therefore, this has clinical significance in terms of appropriateness of prescribing an antidepressant drug, especially in the elderly in whom cardiovascular disease is more prevalent; and, as stated above, 10% of these patients are likely to have bundle branch block. For this reason, several studies have attempted to define the effects of the tricyclic drugs on the heart more completely.

Investigators at the University of Melbourne found that low concentrations of tricyclic drugs led to an anticholinergic action (e.g., increased heart rate) in depressed patients with normal hearts [27]. With increased concentrations, the tricyclics blocked the reuptake of norepinephrine and raised the level of circulating catecholamine in these patients. At higher than therapeutic concentrations, TCAs blocked the action of catecholamine on the heart. This action included prolongation of the HV interval and a wide QRS, indicating prolonged intracardiac conduction. In addition, like quinidine, the tricyclic antidepressants depressed myocardial contractions, heart rate and coronary blood flow. In patients who took fatal overdoses of tricyclics, ECGs showed sinus tachycardia, conduction defects, supraventricular tachycardia, ST and T wave abnormalities, ventricular arrhythmias, profound bradycardia, and asystole [27].

The cardiac function of 32 depressed patients with normal hearts was studied before and during 2 weeks of treatment with nortriptyline, doxepin, imipramine or amitriptyline. Statistically significant increases in heart rate were found in 26 of the 32 patients. The PR interval was increased in all patients [20, 27,

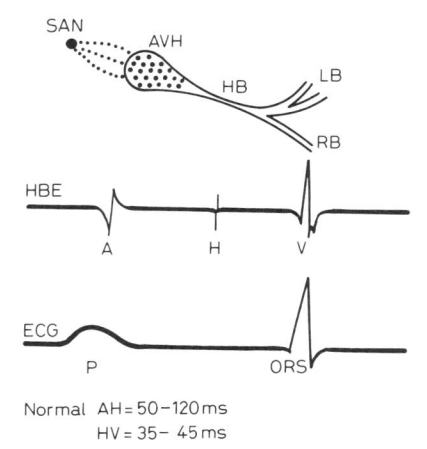

Doxepin: Recent Pharmacologic and Clinical Studies 137

Normal AH = 50-120 ms
HV = 35- 45 ms

Fig. 3. Record obtained by His bundle electrocardiographic technique. Top = Conduction system of the heart; middle = AH and HV interval measurements; bottom = relationship of AH and HV intervals to ordinary ECG. HV interval measures intraventricular conduction time [20].
(Reprinted by permission from B. Davies et al.: "Effects on the heart of different tricyclic antidepressants," in Mendels (ed.), *Sinequan: A Monograph of Recent Clinical Studies.* Amsterdam and Princeton: Excerpta Medica, 1975.)

28]. Since the PR interval usually decreases with increased heart rate, the investigators concluded that the tricyclic drugs prolong atrioventricular conduction.

A follow-up study, using His bundle electrocardiographic techniques [20, 29, 30], evaluated intracardiac conduction in depressed patients taking therapeutic doses of tricyclics. In this method, an electrocatheter is passed via the femoral vein across the tricuspid valve while another electrode is passed into the right atrium (fig. 3). Five of 12 patients treated with daily doses of 150 mg nortriptyline, who had plasma TCA levels over 200 ng/ml, showed a prolonged HV interval. Medication for 1 patient with a markedly prolonged HV interval was then changed to doxepin (at the same dosage). The HV interval returned to normal.

Another study investigated the ECG changes of 14 patients admitted to hospital after tricyclic overdoses [20, 29, 31]: 8 patients were overdosed with amitriptyline, imipramine or nortriptyline; 6 patients were overdosed with doxepin. Of those in the first group, 7 out of 8 showed an abnormal HV interval and widened QRS complex. However, none of the 6 patients overdosed with doxepin showed any change in the HV interval. This indicates normal intracardiac conduction with doxepin.

In a crossover comparison of nortriptyline and doxepin, 34 depressed patients were studied [19]. Half the group received doxepin and the other half received nortriptyline at doses of 150 mg/day; 6 of 17 patients given nortriptyline showed at least 25% prolongation of the QRS complex, while only 1 of 17 patients given doxepin showed this effect. It was concluded that doxepin may be preferable to those tricyclics which can cause ECG abnormalities.

Hayes et al. [32] suggest that some sudden deaths observed in patients who had been on tricyclic antidepressants may be caused by orthostatic hypotension with cardiac ischemia and resultant fatal arrhythmia rather than by direct cardiotoxicity. Their data also indicate that not only geriatric patients, cardiac patients, or overdosed patients are at risk, but all patients receiving tricyclic antidepressants have significant orthostatic hypotension at some phase during early treatment. In a retrospective study conducted by *Glassman* et al. [33], almost 20% of patients receiving an average dosage of 225 mg of imipramine had symptoms associated with orthostatic hypotension severe enough to interfere with their treatment. Over 4% suffered serious physical injuries. We do not know whether this also occurs with doxepin.

Ayd [34] reported that he saw no evidence of any increased risk of hypotensive effects with doxepin therapy in elderly patients. Furthermore, only some elderly patients receiving long-term therapy with doxepin showed transient tachycardia when given doses over 200 mg/day [34]. Doses below this level appeared to cause no adverse cardiovascular effects during 6 or more years of chronic administration.

In a follow-up of 10 years' experience with maintenance doxepin therapy, *Ayd* [35] concludes that long-term doxepin therapy is effective and safe. Of 46 patients (aged 37–75 years), 39 had pretreatment ECGs, 26 of which were normal and 13 abnormal. During doxepin therapy, some patients with pretreatment ECG abnormalities had similar ECG changes throughout doxepin therapy, while in others such pretreatment abnormalities ceased during doxepin therapy [35]. In those patients who developed ECG abnormalities during treatment, ECG changes were either transient or asymptomatic and appeared only at the end of the survey after several years of doxepin therapy.

Doxepin Treatment in the Elderly

In the year 1900, 3% of the American population was over 65 years of age. In 1975, approximately 12% of the population was over 65 years old. The reported incidence of depression in the elderly is increasing. Therefore, the importance of an adequate, well-tolerated dosage, leading to effective antidepressant treatment for patients in this age group, cannot be overemphasized.

Some psychotherapeutic agents are not well tolerated by the geriatric patient. However, doxepin is effective and well tolerated by elderly depressed patients [34, 36]. No abnormal ECG changes attributable to drug treatment were observed in a double-blind placebo-controlled study [37]. Hypotension and tachycardia have a very low incidence following doxepin therapy in the aged [34]. Therefore, doxepin appears to be a particularly suitable drug for depressed geriatric patients.

Because of the increased susceptibility to anticholinergic side effects in the elderly, it is recommended that doxepin treatment be started with a low dose (e.g., 25 mg) at bedtime. It must be stressed, however, that some elderly patients need, and can tolerate, 150–300 mg daily if the dose is gradually increased. At these higher dosage levels, a divided dosage is recommended (giving part with the evening meal and the remainder at bedtime) to minimize the risk of orthostatic hypotension when the patient gets up to void.

Several studies suggest that doxepin has considerably fewer anticholinergic properties than amitriptyline, somewhat fewer than imipramine, and somewhat more than desipramine [8, 39, 40]. This is an important consideration in elderly depressed patients who tolerate side effects such as dry mouth and urinary retention less well than younger patients, and who may be more at risk of developing glaucoma.

Cardiovascular disorders are more common in the elderly. Studies reporting a significant incidence of sudden death among patients with preexisting heart disease taking therapeutic doses of amitriptyline have raised concern about the cardiotoxicity of tricyclic antidepressants [29, 41]. Therefore, every patient, particularly the elderly, should have an ECG before starting tricyclic antidepressant treatment. As noted above, doxepin appears the drug of choice for patients with intracardiac conduction defects. Nonetheless, it must be remembered that overdoses of doxepin, as with other tricyclic antidepressants, disturb the cardiac rhythm.

Sedative and Antianxiety Actions of Doxepin

As noted above, TCAs have antihistaminic properties and may act via the activation of H_1 and H_2 receptors. For any drug, it is difficult to separate a primary anxiolytic effect from a more generalized effect secondary to sedation. The significant sedative potential of doxepin may be responsible for its reported effects in relieving anxiety. Studies using doxepin for the treatment of anxiety used significantly lower daily dosages than recommended for the treatment of depression.

Doxepin may be particularly suitable for moderately anxious depressives because it has antianxiety and antidepressant properties. Both depression and anxiety may produce or exacerbate pain; and while doxepin has not been shown to have analgesic properties per se, it has been reported in preliminary studies that it lowers the need for analgesics among some depressed patients, especially when symptoms of anxiety are also present [40]. These preliminary results are interesting because they may reveal another mechanism of action of doxepin unrelated to its antidepressant effect. Further research is needed in this area before any conclusions can be drawn.

Effect of Doxepin in Patients with Sleep Disturbances

Sleep disturbance is one of the most disabling symptoms of a depressive illness. Classically, this sleep disturbance is described as middle insomnia and early morning awakening (disrupted second and third phases of sleep). Many patients report difficulty in falling asleep. We usually attribute this to the anxiety or agitation components that frequently accompany depression.

The significant clinical advantage of a medication that produces an immediate improvement in sleep pattern is obvious. Most studies have shown significant improvement in the disturbed sleep pattern of depressed patients treated with doxepin. Doxepin significantly increases total sleep time and causes increases in stage three and stage four sleep [41, 42]. Improved electroencephalographic/electrooculographic (EEG-EOG) sleep patterns following doxepin treatment reflect the normalization of sleep patterns in neurotically depressed patients [41]. This parallels improvement of the clinical symptoms of depression [16, 41, 42]. As noted above, doxepin appears to alleviate sleep disturbances by the 1st week of therapy [17]. In the elderly, doxepin is at least as effective as amitriptyline, and superior to both imipramine and desipramine in relieving sleep disturbances.

Practical Considerations

The most important practical considerations in prescribing tricyclic antidepressants are adequate doses and delivery and duration of the therapy. Initial patient workup should include baseline ECG recordings whenever possible. Since TCAs have a wide range of side effects, patient education is often necessary to assure compliance. The risk of side effects, however, should not prevent the physician from slowly increasing the dose to adequate therapeutic levels to achieve a clinical response.

Single daily dose regimens of psychotherapeutic drugs have many advantages. Adverse reactions are less troublesome when plasma TCA levels peak while the patient is asleep. One study reported that qHS medication scheduling led to an improvement in sleep and to a decrease of side effects [37]. Patient compliance decreases markedly when medication is taken in divided doses. Only 50% of patients on a three times daily schedule take their medications in the prescribed manner. Involving a family member in the patient's therapy also results in more reliable delivery of medication.

Conclusions

Doxepin is an effective antidepressant with mood elevating qualities similar to amitriptyline and imipramine. The profile of side effects reported for doxepin is shown in table I. In general, doxepin produces the same side effects as other tricyclic antidepressants. However, it is more sedative and has less an-

Table I. Incidence of side effects from studies analyzed by *Pinder* [38]

Side effect	All patients, % (n = 1,183)[1]	Depressed patients,[2] % (n = 917)[1]	Anxious patients,[3] % (n = 266)
Drowsiness	29.1	28.5	31.2
Dry mouth	27.0	29.1	19.5
Constipation	9.4	10.3	6.4
Dizziness	8.7	7.5	12.8
Extrapyramidal reactions	4.1	3.6	5.6
Blurred vision	3.8	3.8	3.8
Sweating	3.8	3.2	1.9
Hypotension	2.4	3.0	0
Tachycardia	1.7	1.6	1.9

[1] 1,210 for drowsiness; 944 in depressed patients. Some studies recorded other side effects but gave data only for drowsiness.
[2] Includes those with some depression component.
[3] Includes those with some anxiety component.
(Reprinted with permission from R.N. Pinder et al.: "Doxepin: A review of the pharmacologic properties and therapeutic efficacy with particular reference to depression," *Drugs*, Vol. 13, pp. 161–218, 1977; modified with permission of authors and publisher. Sydney, Australia and New York: Adis Press, Ltd.)

ticholinergic activity. This makes it more useful than imipramine in depressed patients who have sleep disturbances, and in depression associated with anxiety. The lower incidence of anticholinergic effects associated with doxepin makes it superior to amitriptyline in those patients, particularly the elderly, who are most at risk. Liquid formulation of doxepin is an alternative dosage form, especially for the aged. At present, doxepin should be considered the antidepressant drug of choice for patients with cardiovascular disease, particularly those with conduction defects. However, as with any tricyclic drug, one should begin with a low dose and titrate the patient up to therapeutic levels with careful ECG monitoring. It should also be remembered that an overdose of doxepin has an intrinsic cardiotoxicity similar to other tricyclic antidepressants.

References

1 Schildkraut, J.J.: Neuropsychopharmacology and the affective disorders (Little Brown, Boston 1970).
2 Glowinski, J.; Axelrod, J.: Effect of drugs on the uptake, release and metabolism of H^3-norepinephrine in the rat brain. J. Pharmac. exp. Ther. *149:* 43 (1965).
3 Tuomisto, J.: A new modification for studying 5-HT uptake by blood platelets. A re-evaluation of tricyclic antidepressants as uptake inhibitors. J. Pharm. Pharmac. *26:* 92 (1974).
4 Frazer, A.: Adrenergic responses in depression. Implications for a receptor defect; in Mendels, Psychobiology of depression, chap. 2, p. 7 (Spectrum, New York 1975).
5 Tehrani, J.B.; Rossi, G.V.; Goldstein, F.J.: Doxepin and imipramine. Effect on catecholamine inhibition of ganglionic transmission. Life Sci. *17:* 257 (1975).
6 Karobath, M.E.: Tricyclic antidepressive drugs and dopamine-sensitive adenylate cyclase from rat brain striatum. Eur. J. Pharmacol. *30:* 159 (1975).
7 Richelson, E.: Tricyclic antidepressants and neurotransmitter receptors. Psychiat. Ann. *9* (1979).
8 Ribbentrop, A.; Schaumann, W.: Pharmakologische Untersuchungen mit Doxepin, einem Antidepressivum mit zentral anticholinerger und sedierender Wirkung. Ärztl. Forsch. *15:* 863 (1965).
9 Ayd, F.J.: Central anticholinergic activity and tricyclic antidepressant efficacy. Int. Drug Ther. Newslett. *10:* 21 (1975).
10 Brunswick, D.J.: Mendels, J.: Reduced levels of tricyclic antidepressants in plasma from vacutainers. Commun. Psychopharmacol. *1:* 131–134 (1977).
11 Kline, N.S.; Cooper, T.; Johnston, B.: Doxepin and desmethyldoxepin serum levels and clinical response; in Gottschalk, Merlis, Pharmacokinetics of psychoactive drugs: Blood levels and clinical response, p. 221 (Spectrum, New York 1976).

12 Friedel, R.O.; Raskind, M.A.: Relationship of blood levels of Sinequan to clinical effects in treatment of depression in aged patients; in Mendels, Sinequan. A monograph of recent clinical studies, p. 51 (Excerpta Medica, Amsterdam 1975).
13 Ward, N.G.; Friedel, R.O.; Bloom, V.L.: The relationship of tricyclic plasma levels to antidepressant response. APA 30th Inst. Hospital and Community Psychiatry, Kansas City 1978.
14 Morris, J.B.; Beck, A.T.: The efficacy of antidepressant drugs. A review of research (1958 to 1972). Archs. gen. Psychiat. *30* (1974).
15 Grof, P.; Saxena, B.; Cantor, R.; et al.: Doxepin versus amitriptyline in depression. A sequential double-blind study. Curr. ther. Res. *16:* 470 (1974).
16 Castrogiovanni, P.; Placidi, G.E.; Maggini, C.; et al.: Clinical investigation of doxepin in depressed patients. Pilot open study, controlled double-blind trial versus imipramine, and all-night polygraphic study. Pharmakopsychiat. Neuro-Psychopharmakopolygraphie *4:* 170 (1971).
17 Mendels, J.; Secunda, S.; DiGiacomo, J.: Depression. An underdiagnosed syndrome? Scientific Exhibit, APA Annual Convention, 1980.
18 Elonen, E.; Mattila, M.J.; Saarnivaara, L.: Cardiovascular effects of amitriptyline, nortriptyline, protriptyline and doxepin in conscious rabbits. Eur. J. Pharmacol. *28:* 178 (1974).
19 Burrows, G.D.; Vohra, J.; Dumovic, P.; et al.: Tricyclic antidepressant drugs and cardiac conduction. Prog. Neuro-Psychopharmacol. (1976).
20 Davies, B.; Burrows, G.D.; Dumovic, P.; et al.: Effects on the heart of different tricyclic antidepressants; in Mendels, Sinequan. A monograph of recent clinical studies, p. 54 (Exerpta Medica, Amsterdam 1975).
21 Fann, W.E.; Cavanaugh, J.H.; Kaufmann, J.S.; et al.: Doxepin. Effects on transport of biogenic amines in man. Psychosomatics *14:* 214 (1973).
22 Oates, J.A.; Fann, W.E.; Cavanaugh, J.H.: Effect of doxepin on the norepinephrine pump. A preliminary report. Psychosomatics *10:* 12 (1969).
23 Gerson, I.M.; Friedman, R.; Unterberger, H.: Non-antagonism of antiadrenergic agents by a dibenzoxepine (Preliminary report). Dis. nerv. Syst. *31:* 780 (1970).
24 American Heart Association: Heart Facts 1979 (American Heart Ass., Dallas 1978).
25 Health United States 1979, US Department of Health, Education and Welfare, Public Health Service Office of Health Research, Statistics and Technology. National Center for Health Services Research, p. 188, US Dept. HEW Publication No. (PHS) 80-1232 (1980).
26 Johnson, R.L.; Averill, K.H.; Lamb, L.E.: Electrocardiographic findings in 67,375 asymptomatic subjects. VII. A-V block. Am. J. Cardiol. *6:* 53 (1960).
27 Burrows, G.D.; Vohra, J.; Hunt, D.; et al.: Cardiac effects of different tricyclic antidepressant drugs. Br. J. Psychiat. *129:* 335 (1976).
28 Vohra, J.; Burrows, G.D.; Sloman, G.: Assessment of cardiovascular side effects of therapeutic doses of tricyclic antidepressant drugs. Aust. N. Z. J. Med. *5:* 7 (1975).

29 Coull, D.C.; Crooks, J.; Dingwall-Fordycee, I.; et al.: A method of monitoring drugs for adverse reactions. Lancet *ii:* 590–591 (1970).
30 Vohra, J.; Burrows, G.D.; Hunt, D.; et al.: The effect of toxic and therapeutic doses of tricyclic antidepressant drugs on intracardiac conduction. Eur. J. Cardiol. *3:* 219 (1975).
31 Vohra, J.; Hunt, D.; Burrows, G.D.; et al.: Intracardiac condition defects following overdose of tricyclic antidepressant drugs. Eur. J. Cardiol. *2/4:* 453 (1975).
32 Hayes, J.R.; Born, G.F.; Rosenbaum, A.H.: Incidence of orthostatic hypotension in patients with primary affective disorders treated with tricyclic antidepressants. Mayo Clin. Proc. *52:* 509–512 (1977).
33 Glassman, A.H.; Giardina, E.V.; Perel, J.M.; Bigger, J.T.; Kantor, S.J.; Davies, M.: Clinical characteristics of imipramine-induced orthostatic hypotension. Lancet *i:* 468–472 (1979).
34 Ayd, F.J.: Maintenance doxepin (Sinequan) therapy for depressive illness. Dis. nerv. Syst. *36:* 109 (1975).
35 Ayd, F.J.: Continuation and maintenance doxepin (Sinequan) therapy. Ten years' experience. Int. Drug Ther. Newslett. *14* (1979).
36 Moser, A.: Doxepin in geriatrics. Med. Hyg. *27:* 1425 (1969).
37 Goldberg, H.L.; Finnerty, R.J.; Cole, J.O.: The effect of doxepin in the aged. Interim report on memory changes and EKG findings; in Mendels, Sinequan. A monograph of recent clinical studies, p. 65 (Excerpta Medica, Amsterdam 1975).
38 Pinder, R.N.; et al.: Doxepin: a review of the pharmacologic properties and therapeutic efficacy with particular reference to depression. Drugs *13:* 161–218 (1977).
39 Peterson, G.R.; Blackwell, B.; Hostetler, R.M.; et al.: Anticholinergic activity of the tricyclic antidepressants desipramine and doxepin in nondepressed volunteers. Communications in psychology, vol. 2. pp. 145–150 (Pergamon Press, New York 1978).
40 Snyder, S.H.; Yamamura, H.I.: Antidepressants and the muscarinic acetylcholine receptor. Archs. gen. Psychiat. *34:* 236–239 (1977).
41 Ward, N.G.; Bloom, V.L.; Friedel, R.O.: The effectiveness of tricyclic antidepressants in the treatment of coexisting pain and depression. Pain *7:* 331–341 (1979).
42 Karacan, I.; Blackburn, A.B.; Thornby, J.I.; et al.: The effect of doxepin HCl (Sinequan) on sleep patterns and clinical symptomatology of neurotic depressed patients with sleep disturbance; in Mendels, Sinequan. A monograph of recent clinical studies, p. 4 (Excerpta Medica, Amsterdam 1975).
43 Karacan, I.; Williams, R.L.; Salis, P.J.: Sleep and sleep abnormalities in depression; in Fann, Karacan, Pokorny, Williams, Phenomenology and treatment of depression, p. 167 (Spectrum, New York 1977).

Discussion

Janowsky: When an adequate dosage of doxepin means a daily dose of 250–300 mg, as it does for some patients, do cardiac effects become more pronounced? Have any studies investigated this?

Secunda: In most studies, the daily dose of doxepin did not exceed 200 mg. However, the Melbourne group studied overdosed patients. They clearly showed that even at toxic levels of the drug (blood levels greater than 300 ng/ml), HV conduction was still normal. This study provides us with a model but epidemiologic studies have not been carried out yet.

Winokur: Orthostatic hypotension is a major problem in TCA therapy because it causes falls, and falls often result in fractures. Elderly patients are particularly susceptible to further complications from fractures. I believe this should be considered when prescribing antidepressant therapy.

Secunda: I agree. I also want to point out that *Glassman* et al. reported that effects of orthostatic hypotension are not dose-related. Maximal effects occur with 75 mg of any of the tricyclics and do not increase with increased dose. Therefore, we must not be afraid of increasing hypotensive effects when our patients require higher doses of a TCA.

Frazer: Tricyclics seem to be the most potent antihistaminic compounds we know. I agree that these antihistaminic properties may be responsible for the sedative effects of doxepin which is the most potent antihistamine of the TCAs. Have you seen other clinical effects that might support this?

Secunda: I have noticed that patients taking doxepin no longer have postnasal drip if that was a problem and, as you might expect, they do not require any antihistamines for other conditions. *Richelson* showed that doxepin has an affinity for H_1 receptors about 800 times that for the commonly used antihistamine diphenhydramine (Benadryl). This confirms my clinical experience.

Mendels: What is known about the pharmacologic and potential clinical activity of the demethylated doxepin?

Secunda: Based on a limited number of studies, it appears that desmethyldoxepin is pharmacologically active. One study suggests that desmethyldoxepin correlates better with therapeutic response than doxepin plus desmethyldoxepin. In animals, desmethyldoxepin is more sedative than doxepin.

Maas: What about studies on plasma levels, response, therapeutic window, etc.? Have any been conducted and, if so, do they add plasma level of doxepin to the demethylated product as is done with imipramine?

Secunda: Yes, the sum of doxepin and desmethyldoxepin is used in determining the therapeutic dose in most studies conducted to date. A therapeutic blood level is reached with values greater than 115 ng/ml. However, *Friedel* studied doxepin and desmethyldoxepin separately. His group suggested that therapeutic response correlates better with the desmethyldoxepin metabolite alone than with either doxepin alone or the sum of doxepin plus desmethyldoxepin. As for the therapeutic window, this seems to correlate with secondary amines not with tertiary amines like doxepin.

The Psychobiology of Affective Disorders. Pfizer Symp. Depression, Boca Raton 1980, pp. 147–165 (Karger, Basel 1980)

Sleep and Circadian Rhythm Disturbances in Depression

David R. Hawkins

Department of Psychiatry, Michael Reese Hospital; Pritzker School of Medicine, University of Chicago, Chicago, Illinois

Sleeping difficulties have been considered one of the hallmark signs of melancholia or depression since the time of Hippocrates. Early morning awakening, moreover, has been identified consistently as a characteristic feature of this disorder. Other characteristic symptoms include rhythm abnormalities, circadian and others, with the diurnal variation from a low point in mood on arising to a high point late in the afternoon or evening being particularly notable. Manics typically sleep little, are not troubled subjectively by sleep loss, and indeed may regard sleep as a waste of time.

It is surprising that until *Aserinsky and Kleitman* [1] discovered the rapid eye movement or REM sleep state, only one group of investigators [2] recognized the value of the electroencephalogram (EEG) in the study of sleep patterns during depressive illness. *Diaz-Guerrero* et al. [2] studied 6 patients under the age of 40, all of whom had been diagnosed as manic-depressive, depressed types. Using the EEG throughout a complete night of sleep, they were able to elucidate correctly the main characteristics of the abnormal sleep pattern found in depressive illness. Although they did not identify the state of REM sleep, they did find that: "The disturbed sleep of patients with manic-depressive psychosis, depressed type, is not only characterized by difficulty in falling asleep and/or by early or frequent awakenings, but by both a greater proportion of sleep which is light and more frequent oscillations from one level of sleep to another than normally occurs."

The following is a brief review of the psychophysiology of sleep and circadian rhythms. A more comprehensive treatment of the subject can be found in *Human Sleep and Its Disorders* [3].

The States of Normal Sleep

NREM Sleep

Normal sleep consists of two states that have profound neurophysiologic differences (fig. 1). The first phase is called nonrapid eye movement, or NREM, sleep. It is also called slow wave sleep (SWS), synchronized sleep (S sleep), or quiet sleep. The sleeper enters this phase initially. Following the onset of NREM sleep, the musculature relaxes although a continuing tonus can be measured by electromyograph. Heart and repiratory rates are slow and regular.

Brain activity, as measured by the EEG, is divided into four stages, generally thought to indicate increasingly less cerebral activity and correlating with increasingly high thresholds for arousal.

In stage 1, which lasts only a few minutes, EEG activity slows from alpha waves, which are 8–12 cycles/second (cps), to beta and theta activity, at 1–6

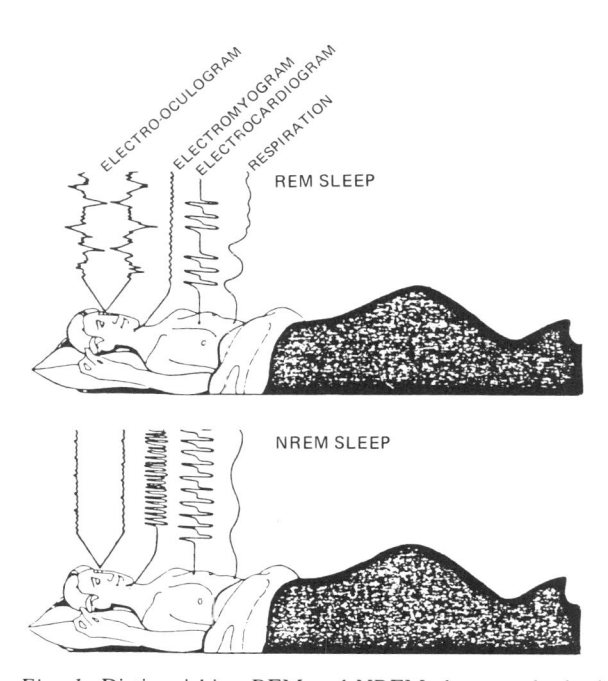

Fig. 1. Distinguishing REM and NREM sleep on the basis of polysomnographic differences [adapted from ref. 40].
(Reprinted by permission from *The Office Guide to Sleep Disorders*, p. 7. KPR Infor/Media Corp., New York, 1980.)

cps. This stage is also characterized by an irregular, low-amplitude, mixed-frequency signal. Slow, rolling eye movements often may be observed.

Stage 2 EEG activity consists, to a large extent, of theta waves with two electrical phenomena present: spindles (12–14 cps waves) and K complexes (which are high-amplitude negative waves followed by positive activity). It is thought that K complexes represent an electrical response to both external and internal stimuli.

Stage 3 sleep is characterized by the presence of slow, high-amplitude delta waves (at 1–4 cps). These delta waves may comprise from 20 to 50% of the EEG record.

Stage 4 is considered the lowest level of physiologic, neurologic, and perhaps psychologic activity. The EEG record shows more than 50% delta waves. The threshold for arousal by external stimuli is higher at this stage than at any other sleep time.

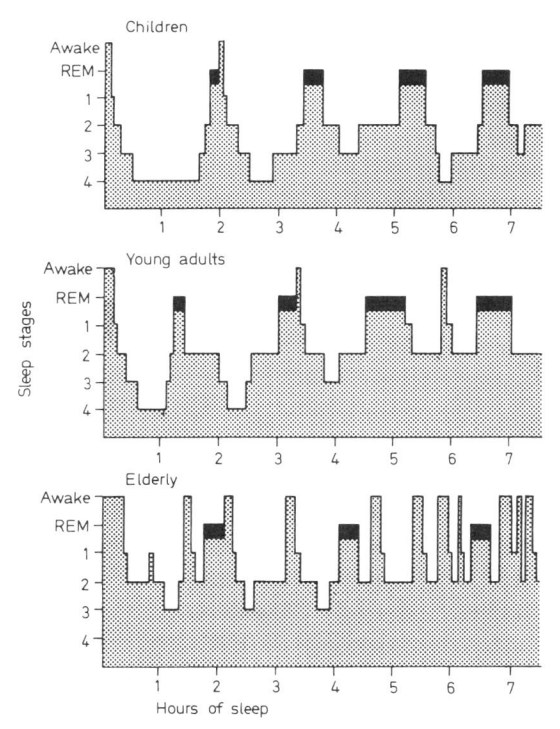

Fig. 2. An idealized night's sleep in children, normal young adults, and the elderly [adapted from ref. 41].
(Reprinted with permission from Anthony Kales: "Sleep and dreams," *Annals of Internal Medicine,* Vol. 68, p. 1081, May 1968).

The approximate distribution of sleep in percentages is: stage 1, 5%; stage 2, 50%; stage 3, 5%; stage 4, 14%; stage 1 REM, 25% [4]. This division of the stages varies at different ages, as shown in figure 2 (stages 3 and 4 are longer in the early part of sleep).

REM Sleep

The second phase of sleep is called rapid eye movement (REM) sleep. Alternative names for this phase are activated, paradoxical, or desynchronized (D) sleep. The REM sleep phase recurs cyclically about every 90 min for 4–6 episodes per night, alternating with NREM sleep. The REM phase begins as the NREM phase ends and the EEG returns to stage 1, as described previously. During this phase, however, there is a complete absence of muscle tone or activity. Brain activity and metabolism increase enormously, matching or even exceeding that of the waking state. Centers in the pons, including the locus ceruleus, control tonic events (increase in brain activity, motor inhibition, and penile erection) and phasic events (burst of rapid eye movements, fine twitching of peripheral musculature, activity of the fine muscles in the middle ear, cardiac and respiratory irregularity).

Under normal circumstances, REM sleep occurs only after more than 45 min of non-REM, or NREM, sleep, and the initial REM period is much shorter than those that follow. When wakened from REM sleep, the subject usually is able to recall a dream with considerable clarity and detail. Using the sleep laboratory, it is possible to selectively deprive a subject of REM sleep. After several nights of such REM deprivation, the percentage of the total sleep period occupied by REM sleep increases to more than the normal 20–25%. Interestingly, after total sleep deprivation for a number of consecutive nights, stage 4 sleep increases, at the expense of all other sleep stages including REM. The obvious implication of these results is that stage 4 sleep is needed more urgently than the other stages, followed by the REM phases.

Sleep and Depression

Early Studies

Sleep laboratory studies of the role of sleep in depression began appearing in the literature in the mid-1960s. These initial studies [5] were cross-sectional, meaning that subjects were studied for 1 or 2 nights in the sleep laboratory at the peak of their depressive illness, or at least as soon as a diagnosis was made. Occasionally, a follow-up study was performed upon recovery.

Difficulties in sleep continuity became apparent in these early studies. Specifically, there was an increased sleep latency (difficulty in falling asleep), increased periods of awakening during the sleep period and, particularly, much more awakening in the latter part of the night (early morning awakening). The most consistent finding was a decrease or absence of delta wave sleep, especially stage 4.

Mean values for REM sleep were found to be decreased. However, the values obtained varied greatly, with some patients actually demonstrating a larger than normal percentage of REM sleep. REM onset latency was found to be shortened. One of the more striking observations when deeply depressed patients were studied was the disruption of the EEG patterning. This disruption was so severe that it was difficult to interpret the sleep records of these patients. Wave patterns not normally seen in juxtaposition frequently were seen side by side in the records of depressed patients. An alpha-delta pattern was observed as well as stage 2 REM sleep.

It became apparent during these early investigations that longitudinal studies were indicated. At present, almost all clinical sleep studies are longitudinal in design. Moreover, they are started now during a drug-free period [6]. Investigators also have been more careful to follow specific diagnostic criteria for affective illness, usually following the criteria established by *Feighner* et al. [7]. A variety of depressive illnesses may appear together in these criteria. Therefore, it is important to remember that differences still may occur between the types of depressive illnesses, and the possibility should be kept in mind that we may still find sleep differences between subgroups. The tendency to overlook this possibility may be a weakness in our investigative efforts to standardize testing.

Sleep Continuity

Kupfer et al. [8] describe sleep continuity as an important feature of sleep studies. In most depressives, there is a sleep onset latency, although this is relatively minor when compared to patients with other disorders, such as some neuroses and primary insomnia.

Most depressives yearn for sleep but are unable to remain in that desirable state. Wakefulness throughout the night has been observed in depressives, although light sleep and frequent awakening occurs much more frequently. The amount of all-night wakefulness increases with more severe cases of depression, and is particularly striking in psychotic patients.

It must be noted, however, that disturbances of sleep continuity are not always present in cases of depression [9, 10]. Some moderately depressed patients actually oversleep; and some patients who have sleep disturbances during severe depressive episodes sleep more than usual when mildly or moderately depressed.

Since clinical observations have indicated that many young depressed patients oversleep, we undertook a study of 20 severely depressed young persons under 26 years of age [11, 12]. On baseline nights, these patients had slightly more wakefulness than matched controls; however, when permitted an extended night of sleep, the depressed patients slept 1½ h longer on average than controls (who also extended their sleep by 1½ h). It is interesting to speculate whether the pattern of oversleeping is an adaptive or protective mechanism in these depressed patients, or if the inability to sleep well later in life plays any role in the etiology or exacerbation of depression. Certainly, an interaction between age and depression has been shown. We know, for example, that depressives over the age of 50 have considerably more abnormal sleep than those under 50 [13].

Sleep Architecture
Sleep architecture refers to the distribution of the various sleep stages [4].

In the depressed individual there are more stage shifts. Also, the regular distinction between stages and the smooth transition from one to another is somewhat disturbed. Typically, there is an increase in the amount of stage 1 and, particularly, stage 2. These two stages represent light sleep. It is thought that the greater increase in stage 2 represents filling in sleep time, caused by the decrease in stages 3 and 4 rather than by a special quality of stage 2 itself. Stage 4, and less often stage 3, seems to be diminished even in young depressed patients who otherwise have shown relatively normal sleep patterns [12].

Even when the depression has been treated successfully, stage 4 sleep is regained much more slowly than all other aspects of normal sleep variables. The diminution of this sleep stage, also called delta wave sleep because of the presence in it of more than 50% delta waves, is not specific to affective illness. It also is seen in the sleep of patients with chronic alcoholism, hypothyroidism, or acute schizophrenia. Delta wave sleep also decreases with age, and it is not known whether this represents a regular linear aging function or whether it is a reflection of possible pathologic changes in the central nervous system.

REM Sleep and Depression
Early sleep laboratory studies of depressed patients focused on the amount of REM sleep. Both increases and decreases in amount were found. In a small

group of patients studied over a prolonged period, without receiving specific therapy, *Snyder* [6] found that REM sleep decreased or increased at different times during the depressive illness. He hypothesized that the increase represented periods in which a rebound effect occurred in order to compensate for a chronic relative REM deficit.

Later studies have shown that REM sleep in depressed patients occurs much earlier after sleep onset than the usual 75–110 min. *Kupfer* [14] has called this shortened REM onset latency a psychobiologic marker for depression. *Kupfer and Foster* [15] have reported that the more severe the depression, the shorter the mean REM latency.

Schulz et al. [16] pointed out that in all previous studies these figures given for REM latency were means and standard deviations. They studied data from 90 polysomnograms of 6 depressed patients and 58 polysomnograms of 4 of these 6 patients after remission. Specifically, they were interested in the frequency distribution of REM sleep latencies. The data revealed two prominent peaks of REM sleep onset, rather than the unimodal distribution common to normal NREM/REM sleep cycle. They concluded that depresserd patients experience an abnormality in regulation of the REM/NREM sleep cycle, with many sleep onset REM phases (SOREMPs), rather than simply shorter REM latency. Occasional SOREMPs also occurred in the depressed patients studied during remission. This fact is significant because SOREMPs are an extremely rare event in normal sleep patterns, and may reflect an alteration in circadian rhythm.

It also has been noted that there is a difference in phasic activity during the REM phase of sleep, as indicated by several measures of eye movement activity. *Kupfer* et al. [8] measured both frequency and intensity of eye movement which they called REM activity (RA). It is higher in depressives than normal subjects, and higher in patients with primary depression compared with those with secondary depresion. *Hauri and Hawkins* [17] used a measure they called percent phasic REM, which correlated negatively with the degree of depression as measured by the Beck Depression Inventory. In sum, in depression there are bursts of eye movements which are more intense than usual, and there are also more and longer times, within a REM period, when there are no actual eye movements.

The length of the initial REM period is another aspect of REM sleep that has received increasing attention [18]. In normal subjects, the initial REM phase is relatively brief. Subsequent phases tend to increase up to approximately four cycles. After this point in the total sleep period, the REM phases begin to decrease [19]. Often, in depressed patients, the initial REM period is long, with subsequent REM periods being shorter. *Vogel* et al. [18] found that in depressed patients the REM periods decrease during many nights, but increase during other nights. This inconsistency again indicates that a shift in the circadian rhythm, or a problem with a postulated sleep cycle oscillator, may occur in depressive illness [18-20].

As to other relationships between sleep and depression, *Hauri* et al. [21] studied 14 formerly depressed subjects, then in clinical remission, in the sleep laboratory and compared their sleep with that of carefully matched controls. All subjects had had at least one episode of primary depression of sufficient severity to require hospitalization, and all had been symptom and drug free for at least 6 months. While their sleep was not strikingly abnormal compared with their controls, they showed increased sleep latency, increased wakefulness and decreased delta sleep. There were fewer interruptions to the REM periods. Within the depressive group, there was more intersubject as well as intrasubject variability of sleep measures. This study suggests that either slight sleep abnormalities are characteristic of those individuals susceptible to depression, or that depressive illness leads to long-lasting abnormalities in the sleep regulatory mechanisms.

The Role of Biochemistry in Depression

Recent evidence indicates that serotonin, norepinephrine, and acetylcholine are necessary for sleep [3]. It is not clear yet whether they influence one of the sleep phases or function as a triggering mechanism. It is also possible that the biogenic amines play a significant role in depressive illness. Investigations in the area of the biochemistry of depression are ongoing, and when the functional relationship of these substances to depression is better understood, we will, presumably, learn a great deal more about the interrelationship between depression and sleep.

The Diagnostic Use of Sleep Studies in Depression

To date, laboratory studies of sleep have not been used clinically for the diagnosis of affective disorders. This is, perhaps, because sleep abnormalities in depression are not sufficiently different from sleep disturbances in other disorders to permit differential diagnosis. *Kupfer and Detre* [22] have reported, however, that, if used within the first days of antidepressant therapy, the sleep laboratory may be useful in predicting which patients will respond well to tricyclic antidepressants. Specifically, when studied during the first 2 nights of treatment, good responders to amitriptyline showed a significant increase in REM latency as well as a decrease in REM sleep percent and activity. These results would indicate that sleep studies may be useful in predicting whether a certain tricyclic drug will be effective.

Manipulation of Sleep as a Therapeutic Tool

It is well known that all the successful antidepressant drugs, with the exception of lithium, have REM-suppressing properties. Based on that knowledge, *Vogel* et al. [23] hypothesized that selective REM deprivation might be effective in a therapeutic sense. In a carefully controlled study, they showed that 17 of 34 endogenously depressed patients responded well to selective REM deprivation. This ratio is equivalent to that expected from treatment with imipramine. It must be noted, however, that reactively depressed patients did not respond to this treatment. At the present time, because REM sleep deprivation therapy is costly and arduous, and no more effective than drug therapy, it does not appear to be clinically applicable.

Pflug and Tolle [24, 25] described another form of sleep deprivation therapy. In their study, patients are deprived totally of sleep for 1 night. This treatment has produced effective results in a significant number of patients. Unfortunately, its effects are not long lasting. It is therefore often combined with antidepressant drugs in the hope that this method will speed the recovery process. The mechanism by which total sleep deprivation works is unknown, but may relate to the interruption it causes in an established abnormal circadian rhythm.

Circadian Rhythm, Sleep and Depression

There are a multitude of cyclic variations in the average human being over each 24-hour period besides the obvious sleep-wake cycle. Activity and arousal levels vary. Body temperature shifts from a high point in the midafternoon to a low point in the early morning hours, several hours before awakening. Studies have shown, in fact, that most biochemical, physiologic, and behavioral functions vary in an organized fashion in normal individuals. This pattern of change is called the circadian rhythm (which means the rhythm of about 1 day).

It is believed that circadian patterns, which are highly precise for each individual, are determined genetically and driven, presumably, by a pacemaker in the central nervous system. This pacemaker has not yet been identified but may consist of multiple self-sustained oscillators that are mutually coupled [20, 26].

Investigators [27] have postulated that the normal endogenous rhythm, which is slightly longer than 24 h, is entrained by various environmental cues, or *Zeitgebers* (a German word meaning "timegivers"). The daily light/dark cycle is the most obvious *Zeitgeber;* however, others, including social phenomena, can entrain an individual's basic diurnal rhythm. This is illustrated by the fact that when animals are studied under artificial lighting conditions, or when humans are isolated from all external cues relating to time or the light/dark cycle (as in underground cave experiments), a regular circadian cycle is still maintained [27].

Some investigators further postulate that more than one circadian rhythm exists in humans. *Kripke* et al. [28] have shown, for example, that at least two separate circadian rhythms of different frequency coexist in humans. Moreover, under certain conditions, the oscillators of the separate circadian rhythms are capable of desynchronizing from each other and/or the external environment.

Sleep Inversion and Circadian Rhythms

Outwardly, humans seem to be able to shift their normal times of sleep abruptly, even so far as to involve a complete sleep inversion or 180° shift in sleep timing. Inwardly, however, most circadian rhythms take up to 2–3 weeks to shift completely and to coordinate normally with activity and sleep.

Weitzman et al. [29] studied 5 healthy young men in the sleep laboratory, reversing their sleep pattern by 180° after a week of baseline measures of their normal sleep rhythm. The results obtained indicate a significant increase in waking and a decrease in REM sleep during the inverted sleep period. The basic 90-min cycling remained intact. Although the number of stage shifts increased, there were no significant changes in the lengths of stages 2, 3, or 4. There were, however, marked decreases in REM latency in many of the subjects studied. Perhaps the most significant change was a shift of REM sleep toward the beginning of sleep and wakefulness toward the end of the sleep period.

These authors point out the similarity of the sleep patterns in this study of complete sleep inversion to those of depressed patients. Both have relatively quick sleep onset, short REM latency, long initial REM periods, and considerable wakefulness at the end of the sleep period. Other studies show that shifts in the timing of sleep lead to dysphoric mood and poor performance, symptoms that remind one of retarded depression [28].

There are many indications that depression, and especially bipolar depression, may be related to abnormal circadian rhythms. Diurnal mood changes, for example, have long been considered characteristic of depression. There also are those patients who cycle regularly between depression and mania.

Beat Phenomena

Halberg [30] proposed that bipolar manic-depressive cycles could result from beat phenomena between body functions that remain synchronized to the 24-hour cycle and others that free run. (The term *beat phenomena* is derived from an analogy to the audible beat produced by two tuning forks of slightly different frequency when the sound waves come at the same instant.) If the two circadian oscillators are desynchronized, there will be times when they come together; that is called the beat phenomena.

Kripke et al. [28] analyzed *Halberg's* [30] proposal that manic-depressive cycles could result from beat phenomena, studying seven manic-depressive patients who had rapid cycles. The patients recorded 3–7 times/day several body functions, including temperature, pulse rate, blood pressure, and finger-counting speed. They also rated their moods at these times on the basis of a 5-point scale.

The results showed that several patients had periods when the shift in their circadian rhythm varied, occurring earlier each day. This suggests that they had oscillators that were free-running at a faster than normal rate. The results obtained from 2 of these patients were particularly interesting in that the predicted beat phenomena corresponded to observed mood cycles. Depression tended to occur when body temperature peaked after midnight, and mania when the temperature peak returned to the late afternoon.

Alterations of Circadian Rhythm

Lithium

It is significant that some circadian rhythms in depressed patients appear to be phase-advanced in their timing. *Kripke* et al. [31] reported studies indicating that lithium slowed circadian rhythms in rodents, cockroaches, and a plant which possessed a prominent circadian rhythm. Accordingly, a study of the effects of lithium on the circadian rhythm in humans was undertaken. Data were collected by the subjects, using sleep logs. In contrast to placebo results, lithium appeared to cause small, but significant delays (14.2 min or 3.64°) in the sleep-wake rhythms.

Elimination of Zeitgebers

Other investigators [32] studied a 66-year-old male patient with 48-hour unipolar depressive cycles during 1 month in a hospital and 2 weeks in an isolation unit, where all *Zeitgebers* were eliminated. The subject alternated regularly between good and bad days. The switch from a normal to a depressive mood invariably occurred during sleep between 10 P.M. and 2:30 A.M. The switch to a good mood was more variable but usually occurred in the afternoon or evening. There was a highly significant correlation on a 24-hour basis between a depressive mood and an increase in urinary free cortisol (UFC). In the isolation unit, there was evidence of internal desynchronization with a rest/activity period of 18.6 h and a period close to 24 h for UFC excretion. While mood changes were associated with both cycles, a close link was demonstrated between the switch from normal to depressive mood and the sleep state.

Sleep Phase Advancement

If some circadian rhythms are indeed phase-advanced in depressed patients, it should be possible to alter the internal phase relationship by advancing the sleep pattern in depressed patients by several hours.

Wehr et al. [33] studied 7 manic-depressive patients longitudinally for evidence of phase shifts and experimentally shifted the sleep phases of several. The patients were monitored continuously for activity by means of a computer-based nontelemetered ambulatory monitor, worn on the nondominant wrist. Plots of motor activity data revealed that 4 of the 7 subjects advanced their time of awakening and activity rapidly as they emerged from the depressive phase of their illness.

One of the patients studied was a 57-year-old woman who had been studied longitudinally for a long period. She had responded to tricyclic antidepressants and sleep deprivation but not to lithium. Her sleep-wake schedule was advanced 6 h on four occasions at approximately 2-week intervals. The initial shift during a depressive episode was from a usual 11 P.M. to 7 A.M. sleep period to a 5 P.M. to 1 A.M. sleep schedule. Two days after the shift, she was in a normal or slightly hypomanic state which lasted 2 weeks.

Her depression remitted again after a further shift to an 11 A.M. to 7 P.M. schedule. Two subsequent 6-hour advances, one as a preventative measure and the other to treat a depressive episode, were unsuccessful for the above patient.

On the first two successful advances, the patient's circadian temperature rhythm advanced. On the other two advances, the temperature rhythm delayed.

It is interesting that during depression, this patient's sleep architecture was typical of a depressive state. After the phase shift, an abrupt trend to normalization occurred, with increasingly normal values seen during periods of complete remission.

In this same study, 2 other depressed patients responded favorably to a phase shift; the last patient's response was equivocal. The authors of this study pointed out that the response to a sleep-wake phase shift is similar to that obtained through sleep deprivation. If it works, the results are immediate. It differs from sleep deprivation in that the improvement lasts longer than 1 day. The results obtained with phase-shift treatment are similar to those obtained with tricyclic antidepressants in that they are relatively long lasting. They differ from tricyclic antidepressants because the results with phase-shift treatment are immediate, while those obtained through use of the drugs take 2–3 weeks.

The number of subjects in this study was too small to permit drawing definite conclusions. Nonetheless, the improvement linked directly to the 6-h imposed advance in the sleep-wake cycle is convincing that positive effects may be derived from this form of therapy. The results also seem to confirm the postulated relationship between altered circadian rhythms and depressive illness.

Biochemical Aspects of Circadian Rhythm

Another study by *Wehr* et al. [34] appeared, again, to confirm the hypothesis that disturbances in central biologic clocks may play a part in the pathophysiology of affective illness. This study was designed to evaluate both the biochemical aspects of neurotransmitter metabolism and the physiologic aspects of circadian rhythm. They studied specifically the circadian rhythm in urinary 3-methoxy-4-hydroxyphenylglycol (MHPG) excretion (which reflects the level of norepinephrine in the brain), motor activity, and oral temperature in 14 normal subjects and 10 manic-depressive patients. The results of the study showed the presence of a daily rhythm in MHPG, with daytime peaks and nighttime nadirs. Compared with the controls, the patients, whether in a depressed or manic phase, showed a shift in the circadian rhythm for each of the measures. This shift ranged from 1 to 3 h earlier than would occur normally. MHPG excretion and motor activity were lower at all times in the depressed patients than in the controls, with the greatest differences occurring in the evening and nighttime samples.

Data from animal studies [35] indicate that hypothalamic norepinephrine may inhibit cortisol production. If MHPG, and hence norepinephrine, is low in depressives early in the night, it would be consistent with the findings of *Sacher* et al. [36] that in depressed patients a higher production of cortisol is most pronounced at night.

A group of investigators in Munich [37] also found an increased secretion of free cortisol in the urine of depressed patients in the early part of the night compared with normal control subjects. In fact, 1 patient exhibited a positive correlation between increased UFC excretion in the first half of the sleep period and the length of the first REM sleep phase.

Those same investigators [38] postulated later that a disturbance in the circadian arousal system accounts for the increased incidence of SOREMPs and also for the resulting bimodal distribution of REM sleep latencies. They further suggest that depressive patients are underaroused during wakefulness and overaroused during sleep. This hypothesis is consistent with those presented by other investigators [39].

Mechanism of Circadian Rhythms in Depression

The evidence is becoming convincing that circadian rhythms are altered in affective disorders in the direction of phase advances and free-running rhythms. Moreover, effective therapeutic agents seem to have the ability to delay circadian rhythm. In at least one instance, advancing the sleep-wake cycle by 6 h was therapeutic.

The major question is: How are the altered rhythms and depression related? Is the alteration in the biologic clock fundamental, or is it just one of the manifestations of a more basic process? If it is fundamental, what triggers the abnormality and what leads to its correction? How do psychologic factors interact with the control mechanisms? Clinically, early morning wakening is seen early in the disease or, at times, without fully developed depression. This seems to represent a need to arouse, to face the unpleasant dangers of the day to come. In this situation, there is often an accompanying urge to get away from the dysphoria of the waking state by going to sleep early. Can this sort of process trigger or upset susceptible internal clocks? Clearly, we are dealing with extremely complicated interrelated mechanisms. The leads, which relate circadian rhythms to the problem of affective illness, are most promising.

References

1 Aserinsky, E.; Kleitman, N.: Regularly occurring periods of eye motility, and concomitant phenomena during sleep. Science *118:* 273–274 (1953).
2 Diaz-Guerrero, R.; Gottlieb, J.S.; Knott, J.R.: The sleep of patients with manic-depressive psychosis, depressive type. Psychosom. Med. *8:* 399–404 (1946).
3 Mendelson, W.B.; Gillin, J.C.; Wyatt, R.J.: Human sleep and its disorders (Plenum Press, New York 1977).
4 Williams, R.L.; Karacan, I.; Hursch, C.J.: Electroencephalography (EEG) of human sleep. Clinical applications (Wiley, New York 1974).
5 Hawkins, D.R.; Mendels, J.: Sleep disturbance in depressive syndromes. Am. J. Psychiat. *123:* 682–690 (1966).
6 Snyder, F.: NIH studies of EEG sleep in affective illness, in Williams, Katz, Shields, Recent advances in the psychobiology of the depressive illnesses (Department of Health, Education and Welfare, Washington 1974).
7 Feighner, J.P.; Robins, E.; Guze, S.B.; et al.: Diagnostic criteria for use in psychiatric research. Archs. gen. Psychiat. *26:* 57–63 (1972).
8 Kupfer, D.J.; Foster, F.G.; Coble, P.; et al.: The application of EEG sleep for the differential diagnosis of affective disorders. Am. J. Psychiat. *135:* 69–74 (1978).
9 Hauri, P.; Hawkins, D.R.: Individual differences in the sleep of depression; in Jovanovic, The nature of sleep, pp. 193–197 (Fischer, Stuttgart 1973).
10 Kupfer, D.J.; Himmelhoch, J.M.; Swartzburg, M.; et al.: Hypersomnia in manic-depressive disease. Dis. nerv. Syst. *33:* 720–724 (1972).
11 Taub, J.M.; Hawkins, D.R.; Van de Castle, R.L.: Electrographic analysis of the sleep cycle in young depressed patients. Psychology *7:* 203–214 (1978).
12 Hawkins, D.R.; Taub, J.M.; Van de Castle, R.L.; et al.: Sleep stage patterns associated with depression in young adult patients; in Koella, Levin, Sleep 1976. Memory, environment, epilepsy, sleep staging (Karger, Basel 1977).
13 Mendels, J.; Hawkins, D.R.: Sleep and depression. A controlled EEG study. Archs. gen. Psychiat. *16:* 344–354 (1967).
14 Kupfer, D.J.: A psychobiologic marker for primary depressive disease. Biol. Psychiat. *11:* 159–174 (1976).
15 Kupfer, D.J.; Foster, F.G.: The sleep of psychotic patients. Does it all look alike? in Freedman, The biology of the major psychoses. A comparative analysis (Raven Press, New York 1975).
16 Schulz, H.; Hurd, R.; Cording, C.; Dirlich, G.: Bimodal distribution of REM sleep latencies in depression. Biol. Psychiat. *14:* 595–600 (1979).
17 Hauri, P.; Hawkins, D.R.: Phasic REM, depression and the relationship between sleeping and waking. Archs. gen. Psychiat. *25:* 56–63 (1971).
18 Vogel, G.W.; Vogel, F.; McAbee, R.S.; Thurmond, A.J.: Improvement of depression by REM sleep deprivation. Archs. gen. Psychiat. *37:* 247–253 (1980).
19 Aserinsky, E.: The maximal capacity for sleep. Rapid eye movement sleep as an index of sleep satiety. Biol. Psychiat. *1:* 147–159 (1969).
20 Hobson, J.A.; McCarly, R.W.; Wyzinski, P.W.: Sleep cycle oscillation. Reciprocal discharge by two brainstem neuronal groups. Science *189:* 55–58 (1975).

21 Hauri, R.; Chernik, D.; Hawkins, D.R.; et al.: Sleep of depressed patients in remission. Archs. gen. Psychiat. *31:* 386–391 (1974).
22 Kupfer, D.J.; Detre, T: Treatment response prediction in affective states. Use of EEG sleep measures. Proc. 11th Coll. Int. Neuro-Psychopharmacol. Congr., Vienna 1978.
23 Vogel, G.W.: Thurmond, A.; Gibbons, P.; et al.: REM sleep reduction effects on depression syndromes. Archs. gen. Psychiat. *32:* 765–777 (1975).
24 Pflug, B.; Tolle, R.: Therapy of endogenous depression by sleep deprivation. Practical and theoretical consequences. Nervenarzt *42:* 117–124 (1971).
25 Pflug, B.; Tolle, R.: Disturbance of the 24-hour rhythm in endogenous depression and the treatment of endogenous depression by sleep deprivation. Int. Pharmacopsychiat. *6:* 187–196 (1971).
26 McCarley, R.W.; Hobson, J.A.: Neuronal excitability modulation over the sleep cycle. A structural and mathematical model. Science *189:* 58–60 (1975).
27 Luce, G.G.: Biological rhythm in psychiatry and medicine. Public Health Service Publication 2088 (United States Government Printing Office, Washington 1970).
28 Kripke, D.F.; Mullaney, D.J.; Atkinson, M., et al.: Circadian rhythm disorder in manic-depressives. Biol. Psychiat. *13:* 335–351 (1978).
29 Weitzman, E.G.; Kripke, D.F.; Goldmacher, D.; et al.: Acute reversal of the sleep-waking cycle in man. Archs. Neurol. *22:* 483–489 (1970).
30 Halberg, F.: Physiologic considerations underlying rhythmometry with special reference to emotional illness; in Ajuriaguerra, Cycles biologiques et psychiatrie (Masson, Paris 1968).
31 Kripke, D.F.; Judd, L.L.; Hubbard, B.; et al.: The effect of lithium carbonate on the circadian rhythm of sleep in normal human subjects. Biol. Psychiat. *14:* 545–548 (1979).
32 Doerr, P.; Von Zerssen, D.; Fischler, M.; et al.: Relationship between mood changes and adrenal cortical activity in a patient with 48 hour unipolar-depressive cycles. J. affect. Dis. *1:* 93–104 (1979).
33 Wehr, T.A.; Wirz-Justice, A.; Goodwin, F.K.; et al.: Phase advance of the circadian sleep-wake cycle as an antidepressant. Science *206:* 710–713 (1979).
34 Wehr, T.A.: Muscettola, G.; Goodwin, F.K.: Urinary 3-methoxy-4-hydroxyphenylglycol circadian rhythm. Archs. gen. Psychiat. *37:* 257–263 (1980).
35 Kreiger, D.T.: Neurotransmitter regulation of ACTH release. Mt. Sinai Med. *40:* 302–314 (1973).
36 Sacher, E.J.; Hellman, L.; Roffwarz, H.P.; et al.: Disrupted 24-hour patterns of cortisol secretion in psychotic depression. Archs. gen. Psychiat. *28:* 19–24 (1973).
37 Schulz, H.; Hurd, R.; Doerr, P.: The measurement of change in sleep during depression and remission. Archs. Psychiat. Nervenkr. *225:* 233–241 (1978).
38 Schulz, H.; Hurd, R.; Cording, C.; et al.: Bimodal distribution of REM sleep latencies in depression. Biol. Psychiat. *14:* 595–600 (1979).
39 Hawkins, D.R.: Depression and sleep research. Basic science and clinical perspectives; in Usdin, Depression. Clinical, biological and psychological perspectives (Brunner/Màzel, New York 1977).

40 Van de Castle, P.L.: Psychology of dreaming (module), p. 27 (General Learning Press, Morristown 1971).
41 Kales, A.: Sleep and dreams. Research on clinical aspects. Ann. intern. Med. 68: 1081 (1968).

Discussion

Dunner: I was under the impression that as people grow older, they sleep less; your data suggest the opposite in controls. Can you explain this?

Hawkins: There are more problems with sleeping as you age. There is a great deal of variation from one individual to another, but certainly older people have increasing difficulty in getting a full night's sleep. There definitely is much more wakefulness. In fact, the sleep of normal older persons in many ways resembles the sleep of depression with wakefulness and with drop-out of stage 4 sleep.

Mendels: There had been suggestions at some time that brain MAO changes with age. Some investigators have speculated that this may be contributing to the reported increased incidence of depression in the elderly.

Dunner: Oscillators actually describe a phenomenon that we do not understand. What mechanism do these oscillators relate to?

Hawkins: It still remains a mystery. The fact that there are biologic clocks has been known for some time. Talk about oscillators is really theoretical. *McCarley and Hobson* in Boston have written extensively on what they conceive of as an "oscillating" mechanism that controls both the switches from REM to non-REM sleep and the shortening and lengthening of REM periods. Mathematical models can be developed that make the possibility of oscillators seem feasible in terms of some of the regulatory functions.

Carroll: When *Kupfer* published his reports a few years ago, we were impressed enough by them to set up a sleep laboratory on our own unit, hoping to use the REM markers in association with our dexamethasone testing. It is interesting that now *Kupfer* is emphasizing the need to take age into account in evaluating the REM-latency figure. He also talks about identifying very young depressives, aged 9 or 10, through REM-latency figures, while you have indicated that they may not apply to young patients. Can you explain this difference of opinion?

Hawkins: We saw no decrease in REM latency in our young depressives and I cannot explain the difference from your reference to *Kupfer's* findings in very young depressives. There is a real question whether we are talking about the same disease we call depression in older persons when we talk about depression in the young. I say that because we had enormous difficulty in finding subjects who would satisfy our criteria for depression. They are depressed, but they do not have the usual symptomatology for depression that we see in older persons. The group we did collect was much more susceptible to mood changes during the day, or from day to day. That raises the question whether we are seeing a different disorder or whether, because of the physiologic or psychologic flexibility of the young, perhaps some sleep-protective mechanisms are operating in this age group that do not in others.

Carroll: We certainly found subjects under the age of 26 who met both RDC criteria and our clinical criteria for endogenous depression, and who also have a high frequency of abnormal dexamethasone testing. Currently, we are looking at their sleep patterns, so in a few more months we might have some other data to deal with.

Hawkins: Are you doing sleep studies?

Carroll: Yes.

Frazer: I would like to comment on the oscillator issue. It is also probable that there are oscillators right in the organs themselves.

Maas: We have done some plasma MHPGs on patients and comparison subjects. We found that there is a steady increase in plasma MHPGs from 8 A.M. to noon; it would therefore appear that a diurnal variation was at play here.

Hawkins: Goodwin and his associates have plotted MHPG and other measures throughout the day, and have found that in both patients and controls daily rhythms for MHPG change.

Lipton: How reliable are the data that indicate that sleep deprivation does affect depression?

Hawkins: There is no question. They have been replicated all over the world now. Clinicians in Europe use it as a means of initial therapy when a patient is going to be treated with antidepressant medication. It is hard to predict for which patient sleep deprivation will work. Also, it is a temporary effect. The typical response is an improvement for a day or two and then a relapse into the depression.

Lipton: Goodwin commented that this might conceivably be looked at as a sort of attempted biologic self-therapy: that the insomnia of depression may be an attempt to heal oneself. First, could you comment on that, and, second, which circadian rhythms are affected? Is anything known at all about whether this results in an alteration in mood?

Hawkins: Goodwin's notion is very interesting but, at this point, purely speculative. Various factors are altered in depression, but which one is the key and clearly related to the illness is not known. When depression is treated by phase advance, it is hoped that all kinds of rhythms may be brought back into synchrony. Which ones, and why, is still far from known.

Mendels: As I understand it, sleep deprivation is an antidepressant, but as you point out, it is temporary, lasting only for a day or two. The question is what evidence might there be that the combined use of tricyclic drugs and sleep deprivation will reduce the latency to antidepressant effect usually seen with tricyclics? This would mean that you help patients right away with deprivation therapy, then the tricyclic will take over and hold them there. Is that an established approach?

Hawkins: It is apparently a widespread practice, and the rationale is that you make the patient feel better somewhat earlier on. I do not think it gets you to the end point any faster. There is some evidence that response to sleep deprivation is another predictor of who will respond favorably to tricyclics.

Carroll: I want to make a point for the general clinician. One of the conclusions of *Kupfer's* group is that the sleep laboratory could be useful in identifying individuals diagnosed as depressive, but who, in fact, have a medical condition underlying their symptoms. These can be a significant proportion of new cases of depression, and it is important to pick them out. Do you have any experience that would verify that?

Hawkins: The average depressed patient has obvious sleep problems. You can make the diagnosis and treat the condition. Unless the sleep laboratory is able to be much more specifically predictive than at the present time, it probably is not of general practical use. On the other hand, the sleep laboratory can be of great value picking up other sleep problems. Most depressions secondary to a medical problem should be clinically obvious. However, if you have a patient who seems depressed and is not responding, sleep laboratory testing is one way of determining whether a medical condition is involved.

Translation of Psychiatric Research into Clinical Practice

George Winokur

Department of Psychiatry, University of Iowa College of Medicine, Iowa City, Iowa

Researchers and clinicians have a lot to gain from one another. It is no secret, however, that some researchers and some clinicians regard each other warily. These researchers consider clinicians dogmatic and opinionated. Some clinicians, on the other hand, believe researchers are impractical and do not understand the compromises that must be made in patient management. Nonetheless, the fact remains that neither the clinician nor the researcher can make therapeutic advances without the other. The clinician, constantly confronted with problems, may suggest viable ideas to the researcher. The researcher may generate new data which the clinician can use in everyday practice. While the pursuit of truth as a goal in itself is a leisure-time activity, research definitely has a practical and salutary influence on clinical care, if only in the long run. That basic and applied research have advanced clinical practice can be documented easily.

There is a hierarchy of research methodologies which is relevant to the clinician. At the top of this hierarchy is clinical research, which includes follow-up studies and short- and long-term drug trials. Next are the genetic and epidemiologic studies which also can be translated into clinical practice. Clinical laboratory research follows. Measurement of tricyclic blood levels and determination of dexamethasone suppression are beginning to show the usefulness of applying laboratory research results to psychiatric practice. Basic applied research, performed in the laboratory on problems clearly related to clinical areas, is next on the list. It includes research with an animal model of depression and attempts to reverse such depressions with various therapeutic interventions. Finally, there is basic nonapplied research which usually poses the greatest difficulty for clinicians. They often see no particular connection between clinical medicine and the events occurring in the laboratory. Nevertheless, there clearly is enormous potential for laboratory research to be relevant to clinical care. In this paper we will explore some aspects of this hierarchy and attempt to document the usefulness of research to the clinician.

Clinical Research

This category contains many findings which are translated into clinical care. For example, table I shows a group of postpartum manic patients who were compared with a matched control group of manic patients and also with a consecutive series of women with mania [1]. Postpartum manics clearly show more evidence of delusional thinking (Schneiderian symptoms) and are less likely to have first-degree relatives with affective illness.

An important finding, in terms of clinical practice, occurred in a follow-up study. In a 3-year follow-up, the postpartum manics experienced no recurrences of mania outside the postpartum period, while in the matched control group six episodes of mania occurred ($p < 0.05$). What practical significance do these results have for the clinician? First, it seems that for a patient with a postpartum mania, and no other manic episodes, long-term lithium prophylaxis may be inappropriate. Second, since postpartum mania frequently recurs with subsequent births, sound treatment for a patient who has had one episode of postpartum mania may be to administer lithium immediately upon delivery and to maintain the patient on lithium for a period of 3 months. This might prevent a sub-

Table 1. Postpartum manics vs. non-postpartum women with mania [1]

	Postpartum manics	Matched control female manics	All female manics except those postpartum
n	21	21	136
Schneiderian symptoms, %	62	—	28*
Follow-up (3 years), recurrence of non-postpartum episodes	no episodes	6 episodes †	—
Subsequent postpartum episodes	one	none	
Number with an affectively ill first-degree relative, %[1]	19	38	36

[1] Differences not significant.
* $\chi^2 = 8.08$, f.d. = 1, $p < 0.005$; † $\chi^2 = 4.86$, d.f. = 1, $p < 0.05$.

sequent manic episode. The patient need not be given lithium indefinitely, as she would be unlikely to have other episodes of mania, with or without lithium, outside the postpartum period.

Another example of clinical research, which can be translated into clinical practice, is shown in the mortality studies described in table II. This large study examined the 1-year mortality for hospitalized depressed patients age 50 or more [2]. Mortality from all causes (i.e., suicide, accident, disease) was included.

Table II. Year mortality for depressed patients aged 50 years or older [2]

	n	Number deceased	% mortality
Total, adequate treatment	212	5	2.4
Total, inadequate treatment	103	11	10.6

Difference between groups $\chi^2 = 8.30$, d.f. $= 1$, $p < 0.005$.

The percent mortality among patients receiving inadequate antidepressant treatment was much higher than that among patients receiving adequate antidepressant treatment ($p < 0.005$). Adequate treatment consisted of electroconvulsive therapy (ECT) or at least 1 month of tricyclic antidepressant (TCA) therapy at a daily dose of 150 mg or more for 2 weeks. Criteria for adequate treatment with monoamine oxidase inhibitors were also given. Inadequate treatment consisted of pharmacotherapy in lower doses than noted above, no ECT, or no antidepressant medication at all. No difference in mortality rates was found between patients receiving adequate TCAs and those given ECTs [2]. The majority of the patients in this study met the research criteria for depression. These data indicate the importance of treating depressed hospitalized patients with adequate antidepressant therapy, using either TCAs or ECTs, in the hope of preventing death within 1 year [2].

Genetic and Epidemiologic Studies

The relevance of genetic and epidemiologic studies to clinical care is easily assessed. Table III shows a study conducted in the Helsinki University Central Hospital on the incidence of suicides, at various periods throughout this century, in depressed hospitalized patients [3].

Table III. Suicides in the Department of Psychiatry of Helsinki University Central Hospital at various periods [3]

	1921–1950	1951–1960	1961–1971
Number treated	13,192	7,579	9,505
Number of suicides	11	8	21
Proportion suicides, %	0.08	0.11	0.22
Suicides of all deaths, %	2.0	17.0	66.0

The period 1921–1950 is characterized by the relative restriction of inpatient activities and the introduction, in 1937, of ECT. The wide use of electroconvulsive therapy in that hospital continued until the 1950s. The period 1951–1960 was characterized by increased use of pharmacologic agents and decreased use of ECT in the treatment of depression. In the period 1961–1971, milieu therapy and increased freedom of inpatient activities were introduced. Strikingly, the incidence of suicides in the hospital rises in each succeeding period. Suicides account for more and more hospital deaths as time goes on. This study implies that although many clinicians are reluctant to use it, severely depressed patients admitted to hospital may benefit from ECT. It may be of some significance for the clinician to consider this form of therapy for potentially suicidal patients.

Table IV illustrates another example of the use of epidemiologic research in evaluating treatment for depression. This study assessed mortality in hospitalized psychiatric patients in Norway [4]. In the period 1950–1962, ECT reached its peak as the treatment of choice for depression. In the period 1963–1968, drug therapy became the treatment of choice. This latter period

Table IV. Excess mortality for unnatural deaths (nonorganic causes) of psychotics who died in psychiatric hospitals [4][1]

	1950–1962	1963–1974
Number of unnatural deaths, men	145	370
Excess mortality, observed/expected	1.6	3.4–4.5
Number of unnatural deaths, women	57	167
Excess mortality, observed/expected	3.3	8.1–9.3

[1] 56–63% of male deaths and 44–45% of female deaths were suicides.
30–41% of male deaths and 52–54% of female deaths were accidents (mostly fractures, some intoxications)

was also characterized by the introduction of more liberalized ward policies and milieu therapy. Unnatural deaths (from suicide, fractures, or intoxications) were markedly increased in this period.

Increased mortality in these studies probably reflects changes in the treatment of depression. It is interesting to note that not all deaths resulted from suicides. A large percentage were owing to accidents, mostly fractures and intoxications. We know from the data of *Glassman* et al. [5] that nearly 20% of depressed patients treated with imipramine have orthostatic hypotension. Orthostatic hypotension, especially among elderly patients, can lead to falls and fractures. If we assume that some patients in the Norwegian study received imipramine therapy, this could account for some of the unnatural deaths. How can the clinician make use of such data? First, they indicate the need for administering either those tricyclic antidepressants which cause little or no orthostatic hypotension, or the possibility of using other antidepressant treatments, such as ECT, in those patients most at risk from this side effect. Furthermore, in depressed patients with known bone fragility or bone disease (the Norwegian study probably reflects the increased incidence of osteoporosis among Scandinavian women), these data indicate that ECT might be an appropriate form of antidepressant treatment.

Table V illustrates an example of a genetic study which affords practical information to the clinician. In a blind evaluation of the families of 28 acute (schizoaffective) and 25 chronic schizophrenics, investigators found that familial schizophrenia is more common in the families of chronic schizophrenics and affective disorder is more common in the families of acute schizophrenics [6]. This indicated that acute schizophrenia (synonyms: schizoaffective illness, good prognosis schizophrenia, good premorbid schizophrenia, schizophreniform illness, reactive psychosis, cycloid psychosis, psychogenic psychosis, atypical psychosis) is related closely to affective disorder. It also indicated that lithium treatment might be useful in such patients. When studies using lithium therapy were conducted with schizoaffective patients, they responded well

Table V. Family background in acute vs. chronic schizophrenics (primary relatives, blind diagnosis)

Morbidity risk for	Chronic schizophrenics, % (n = 25)	Acute schizophrenics, % (n = 28)
Familial schizophrenia	15.1	5.5
Familial affective disorder	4.5	20.1

to this treatment [7]. They also responded well to ECT [8]. Such family studies help clarify clinical issues for the practicing psychiatrist.

Clinical Laboratory Research

Clinical laboratory research is the frontier of psychiatric research at the present time. An example of its potential usefulness is illustrated by the dexamethasone suppression test. *Carroll* et al. [9] have shown that a large proportion of unipolar depressives exhibit abnormal nonsuppression of serum cortisol when given dexamethasone the previous night.

In a study reported by *Schlesser* et al. [10], 1 mg of dexamethasone was administered at 11 P.M., blood samples were collected at 8 A.M. the next morning, and cortisol determinations were made. Table VI shows the results of this study in unipolar depressives and in controls. Almost half of the unipolar depressives had an abnormal response to the dexamethasone challenge. What is the practical significance of such findings? When a diagnosis of affective illness is questionable, the dexamethasone suppression test sometimes proves useful. While a normal response does not rule out the possibility of affective disorder, an abnormal response is highly suggestive of this type of illness. Also, the dexamethasone suppression test may be useful in monitoring treatment results since it appears to be state-dependent and to revert to normal on improvement.

Table VI. Abnormal dexamethasone nonsuppressors (>5 µg/dl) in unipolar depression

Diagnosis	n	Proportion nonsuppressors
Unipolar depression	86	43%
Manics	45	0
Schizophrenics	35	0

Similarly, *Kirkegaard and Bjørum* [11] published clinical laboratory data in 35 patients with endogenous depression showing that the changes in the peak thyroid-stimulating hormone (TSH) response to thyrotropin-releasing hormone (TRH) might be prognostic in predicting early relapse. Patients in this study were given 200 mg TRH intravenously, and TSH was measured. The patients were then treated with ECT until they obtained clinical recovery, and the TRH test was repeated. Patients were followed, without antidepressant therapy, for 6

Table VII. TSH response (Δ max TSH) to TRH in endogenous depression

		% relapses
<2.0 μU/ml	19	100
>2.0 μU/ml	16	19

months or until they relapsed (table VII). All of patients who had a TSH response to TRH lower than 2.0 μU/ml, after ECT, relapsed. In contrast, only 19% of patients who had a response to the TRH test greater than 2.0 μU/ml, after ECT, relapsed. Thus, this test may prove to have clinical usefulness in the future.

Basic Applied Research

Basic applied research deals primarily with laboratory research that is clearly related to clinical problems. Animal models of psychiatric illnesses fit this category. The learned helplessness model of depression, which may have some relevance to psychopharmacology, is a good example. *Sherman* et al. [12], *Petty and Sherman* [13, 15] and *Sherman and Allers* [14] reported that the behavioral state induced by learned helplessness could be prevented or reversed by antidepressants but not by other types of psychotropic drugs. They demonstrated a significant effect after only 4 days of TCA administration. Tricyclic antidepressants elevated hippocampal levels of the demethylated metabolites beyond an effective level of 1.65 μg/g. Secondary amine metabolites of TCAs, but not the parent compounds, were effective in preventing development of learned helplessness. Injection of gamma-aminobutyric acid (GABA) or desipramine into the anterior neocortex, hippocampus, or lateral geniculate body, as well as injection of norepinephrine into the hippocampus, produces similar prophylactic effects. Each of these treatments prevents a decrease in neocortical levels of 5-hydroxyindoleacetic acid, suggestive of an interaction with the serotonergic system.

The studies described above may have some clinical usefulness. They may, in the long run, help us to better understand the pathophysiology of depression and to develop new and more effective phramacologic agents for the treatment of this disorder. After more data have been gathered, perhaps clinicians will be able to use these findings and modify clinical practice accordingly.

Basic Nonapplied Research

Many basic nonapplied research studies involve neurochemistry. An example is the study of mammalian astroglial cells which may play a fundamental role in the central nervous system [16–22]. *Henn and Hamberger* [16] initially described GABA uptake by astrocytes, and further research on several other neurotransmitters has shown that astroglia may contribute to the extracellular concentration of amino acids. Also, astrocytes can regulate the extracellular concentration of ions such as potassium. Therefore, astrocytes may also regulate the concentrations of some extracellular components critical to neuronal activity. *Henn* [17] recently reported that astroglia have receptors for dopamine and benzodiazepines. This finding suggests that receptors mediating neuroleptics and antianxiety drugs might act through astroglial cell alterations. This, in turn, suggests that astroglial cells interact with psychotropic agents which would alter metabolic patterns affecting neuronal function. Experimental work supports this concept in the case of neuroleptics and schizophrenia [16–22]. There may be other receptors on astroglia relevant to antidepressant drugs. At present, this work cannot be applied to clinical practice. However, with further research it may prove useful to the psychiatrist.

Discussion

Over the past few decades, psychiatric research has greatly advanced the practice of psychiatry. Not only the advent of psychopharmacology but also its improved practice came about from research studies. For example, data on the half-life of drugs, on adequate dosage regimens, and on possible side effects have substantially changed clinical practice and the management of depressed patients. The substantial reduction in the number of patients hospitalized for clinical depression probably reflects the more effective and appropriate use of psychopharmacology by clinicians. While these results are well incorporated into psychiatric practice today, other findings are incorporated more slowly. Therefore, it may be difficult, at the present time, to understand and translate the implications of some of the studies reviewed in this paper in terms of clinical applicability. Nonetheless, the evidence suggests that at least some will prove to have clinical significance.

Overall, great strides have been made in psychiatric practice as a result of well-controlled clinical research studies. Clinicians and researchers both play important roles in these advances. The potential for fruitful interaction is obvious, especially now when increasing numbers of psychiatric research studies are beginning to be conducted on outpatients.

References

1 Kadrmas, A.; Winokur, G; Crowe, R.: Postpartum mania. Br. J. Psychiat. *135:* 551–554 (1979).
2 Avery, D.; Winokur, G.: Mortality in depressed patients treated with electroconvulsive therapy and antidepressants. Archs. gen. Psychiat. *33:* 1029–1037 (1976).
3 Lönnqvist, J.; Niskanen, P.; Rinta-Mänty, R.; et al.: Suicides in psychiatric hospitals in different therapeutic eras, a review of the literature and own study. Psychiat. Fenn. 265–273 (1974).
4 Fegersten Saugstad, L.; Ødegard, Ø.: Mortality in psychiatric hospitals in Norway, 1950–74. Acta psychiat. scand. *59:* 431–447 (1979).
5 Glassman, A.; Biggs, J.T.; Giardina, E.; et al.: Clinical characteristics of imipramine-induced orthostatic hypotension. Lancet *i:* 468–472 (1979).
6 McCabe, M.; Fowler, R.C.; Cadoret, R.; et al.: Familial differences in schizophrenia with good and poor prognosis. Psychol. Med. *1:* 326–332 (1971).
7 Perris, C.: Morbidity suppressive effect of lithium carbonate in cycloid psychosis. Archs. gen. Psychiat. *35:* 328–331 (1978).
8 Avery, D.; Winokur, G.: The efficacy of electroconvulsive therapy and antidepressants in depression. Biol. Psychiat. *12:* 507–523 (1977).
9 Carroll, B.; Curtis, G.; Mendels, J.: Neuroendocrine regulation in depression. II. Discrimination of depressed from non-depressed patients. Archs. gen. Psychiat. *33:* 1051–1058 (1976).
10 Schlesser, M.; Winokur, G.; Sherman, B.: Genetic subtypes of unipolar primary depressive illness distinguished by hypothalamic-pituitary-adrenal axis activity. Lancet *i:* 739–741 (1979).
11 Kirkegaard, C.; Bjørum, N.: TSH responses to TRH in endogenous depression. Lancet *i:* 152 (1980).
12 Sherman, A.D.; Allers, G.L.; Petty, F.; et al.: A neuropharmacologically relevant animal model of depression. Neuropharmacology *18:* 891–893 (1979).
13 Petty, F.; Sherman, A.D.: Reversal of learned helplessness by imipramine. Commun. Psychopharmacol. (1980).
14 Sherman, A.D.; Allers, G.L.: Relationship between regional distribution of imipramine and its effect on learned helplessness in the rat. Neuropharmacology (1980).
15 Petty, F.; Sherman, A.D.: Regional aspects of the prevention of learned helplessness by desipramine. Life Sci. (submitted for publication).
16 Henn, F.A.; Hamberger, A.: Glial cell function. Uptake of transmitter substances. Proc. natn. Acad. Sci. USA *68:* 2686–2690 (1971).
17 Henn, F.A.: Neurotransmission and glial cells. A functional relationship? J. Neurosci. Res. *2:* 271–282 (1976).

18 Henn, F.A.; Haljamäe, H.; Hamberger, A.: Glial cell function. Active control of extracellular K⁺ concentration. Brain Res. *43:* 437–443 (1972).
19 Franck, G.; Grisar, T.H.; Moonen, G., et al.: Potassium transport in mammalian astroglia; in Schoffeniels, Granck, Towers, Hertz, Dynamic properties of glial cells (Pergamon Press, London 1978).
20 Henn, F.A.; Anderson, D.J.; Sellstrom, A.: Possible relationship between glial cells, dopamine and the effects of antipsychotic drugs. Nature, Lond. *266:* 637–638 (1977).
21 Henn, F.A.; Henke, D.: The cellular localization of dopamine receptors. Neuropharmacology *17:* 985–988 (1978).
22 Henn, F.A.: Relationship of GABA and diazepam receptors in cerebellar purkinje cells. Brain Res. Bull., suppl 2 (1980).

Discussion

Katz: You singled out the decreased use of ECT as a major factor associated with increased mortality rates in the Helsinki study. Could there be other factors as well?

Winokur: Yes. Another factor must be considered. That is, the liberalization of ward policies for inpatients. Both this and the decreased use of ECT may play a role in the increased mortality observed. It is interesting here that no other epidemiologic study with which I am familiar so clearly shows the practical application of research to the clinician.

Carroll: I think it is difficult for many clinicians to match the clinical syndrome with the biochemistry involved in a particular disorder. Researchers must try to bridge this gap.

Winokur: One way of dealing with this problem is by providing in-training conferences for residents where research papers are reviewed critically. Another way is by involving clinicians already in practice in areas of current research. This helps the practicing psychiatrist to evaluate information more critically as well as to participate in data gathering.

Hawkins: One point on which clinicians and researchers appear to diverge seems to me to be on the issue of diagnosis. The Research Diagnostic Criteria, for example, exists for research purposes. It enables us to compare exactly the same type of patient population from one study to the next. However, if a clinician tries to use the RDC, particular patients may not fit neatly into one category or another. This sometimes creates problems. The patient does not fit the criteria, but the physician thinks he or she does and wonders how to treat the patient.

Winokur: I disagree. The Research Diagnostic Criteria cannot be all inclusive, but it is useful in describing a clinical picture. It is inconceivable to me that a depressed patient would not meet the RDC or the Feighner criteria. Of course, there are a number of different kinds of depression within those criteria.

Maas: My experience has been that workers in clinical research are often reluctant to see their findings translated into practical applications because they are aware of all the associated problems. For example, I get many referrals for measuring MHPG levels but I discourage this. There are too many complexities involved in obtaining complete 24-hour urine collections.

Gershon: I am not sure about that. I would be pleased to see clinicians carry out some assays in the hope of better understanding their practical value. Of course, these would have to be done carefully and correctly. I would include radioreceptor assays for phenothiazine, neuroleptics, and dopamine. As long as the assay is done properly, I think MHPG levels should be measured. We cannot use monoamine oxidase as a genetic marker, but, if the assay were available, we would be able to assess dosage levels more accurately when prescribing monoamine oxidase inhibitors. Finally, I think we have to expand the use of reliable drug assays for pharmacokinetic measurements. All these studies would help us advance clinical psychiatric practice.

Winokur: I would like to make a final comment. I want to emphasize that by proceeding with research data we modify our clinical practice as we gain new knowledge. Clinicians frequently pose the questions and researchers search for the answers. There is no question that clinical psychiatric practice has benefited from research. Certainly, we have a good example of this. The substantial change in the treatment of depressed patients and the decreased number of patients who need hospitalization for depressive illness reflects the results of clinical research in psychopharmacology. Clinical research, with all its limitations, is useful and has advanced the field of psychiatry for the clinician.

New Vistas: Depression Research Excluding Norepinephrine, Serotonin, Neuroendocrinology, Cholinergic Systems, and Genetics

Morris A. Lipton

Biological Sciences Research Center, University of North Carolina School of Medicine, Chapel Hill, North Carolina

The title and placement of this presentation, at the end of the program, make it clear that its task is not to recapitulate, but to attempt to examine some areas of ignorance, to look at some new ways of ordering and integrating the existing data (for the purpose of better understanding and treating the affective disorders), and to predict, perhaps, what new insights we might envisage when we complete those studies currently under investigation. Finally, although our overall topic is the Psychobiology of Affective Disorders, the other authors primarily stressed biology. I shall, therefore, emphasize the psychology of depression and its implication for treatment. It must be obvious, however, that a discussion of the psychobiology of depression is impossible without some mention of the wealth of information developed over the past decade on transmitters, receptors, hormones, and genes.

Biologic Considerations

Our hypotheses about the biology of depression derived largely from the study of hospitalized patients with the most severe and usually endogenous depressions. This strategy is good since severely depressed patients usually need hospitalization and can be studied in this controlled environment. Also, we can employ invasive techniques more freely in these patients than in ambulatory patients, and inpatients require pharmacologic agents. From the biochemical actions of such agents, correlated with the clinical responses they engender, we developed most of our hypotheses regarding the pathogenesis and pathophysiology of the affective disorders. But, even with such patients, there remain significant gaps in our knowledge. The drugs we typically employ are not absolutely specific for each neurotransmitter; their acute effects, which have been studied for so long, are quite different from their chronic effects. As *Hartman* [1] has shown, these drugs even have significant effects on the permeability of the small blood vessels of the brain.

All clinical researchers know that inferences about pathobiology derived from successful therapies are much weaker than those derived from interventions that produce illness. The pharmacologic production of depression has been only partially successful. Thus, we are left with conceptual problems. For example, reserpine has long been known to cause depression in about 15–20% of patients receiving this antihypertensive treatment for many months. Close to 100% of hypertensive patients treated with reserpine obtain significant and prolonged relief; 20% of these patients develop depression. Why should 80% of patients be protected from the depressive actions of reserpine while they respond to its antihypertensive action?

The same problem is reflected in the mood changes associated with alpha-methylparatyrosine, a specific catecholamine depletor used in the treatment of pheochromocytoma. Parachlorophenylalanine, a serotonin depletor used in the treatment of carcinoid, also shows similar effects on mood. Patients receiving these drugs improve physically but sometimes show mild mental changes. They may become anxious or lethargic, although typically not depressed. All three drugs diminish peripheral amines. Is the central nervous system of most individuals somehow protected from depletion or, alternatively, can most persons have depleted central nervous system amines and still not get depressed? We simply do not know. We probably will not know until we have more, noninvasive techniques that permit strong inferences about brain events. For example, plasma studies of 3-methoxy-4-hydroxyphenylglycol (MHPG), a specific marker for brain norepinephrine metabolism, in patients who receive reserpine or alpha-methylparatyrosine may differ significantly in patients who become depressed versus those who do not.

It is also clear that we still fail to understand why a long lag exists between achievement of adequate blood levels of the tricyclic antidepressants and a significant clinically therapeutic response. Recently, *DiMascio* et al. [2] studied the rate and degree of differential symptom reduction produced by 100–200 mg/day of amitriptyline in acutely depressed patients. These were ambulatory, neurotic depressives, according to DSM II, and major depressives according to the Research Diagnostic Criteria and DSM III. The patients were neither psychotic nor bipolar, and results cannot be generalized to these groups. The most rapid effect of the drug was on improvement of sleep disturbance. This occurred within a week. The effects on anxiety, depression, and apathy occurred in about 12 weeks. The same study examined symptom reduction with psychotherapy and, interestingly, the main effect of psychotherapy was on anxiety, depression, and apathy with improvement occurring in 1–4 weeks. Reduction in vegetative symptoms took longer. Other studies, using different drugs and higher dosages, have produced more rapid symptom reduction. However, under any circumstances, most depressive symptoms require a few weeks' treatment before clinically significant changes occur. This is substantially longer than the time required for the acute effects of the tricyclics to inhibit inactivation of neurotransmitters by reuptake. It does, however, correlate better with the time required for alteration of receptor sensitivity by alteration of receptor numbers. This process involves protein synthesis and degradation, is not instantaneous, and takes 1–2 weeks.

Sleep is still another area in which we are only beginning to acquire information of both practical and theoretical interest. As *Hawkins* [3] has shown, sleep is grossly distorted in depression. Sleep deprivation has long been considered an unfortunate consequence of depression and its associated insomnia. It is, therefore, surprising to find that purposeful sleep deprivation alone causes a transient relief from depression. When used with tricyclics, sleep deprivation accelerates the rate of recovery from depression [4, 5]. The effectiveness of this therapy in endogenous depressions seems unquestionable, although its mechanism is not understood. It raises the question whether the insomnia of depression is merely an unfortunate symptom or an attempt at self-healing. Several chronobiologic hypotheses have been proposed to explain the improvement in depression following sleep deprivation. Biologic rhythms in neurophysiology and neuroendocrinology are areas of investigation which undoubtedly will receive considerably more attention in the near future.

Finally, there are recent findings about the effect of the administration of pituitary hormones to patients with primary affective disorders. *Gold* et al. [6] in a double-blind placebo-controlled trial, administered a vasopressin congener to 4 patients with major primary affective illness. They found highly significant and consistent improvements in tests designed to measure the formation, coding, and organization of long-term trace events in memory. Two of the patients also showed a significant amelioration of other depressive symptoms. The improvement in cognitive performance of these depressed patients, following vasopressin administration, suggests that there may be a biologic substrate for the impaired cognition of depressives. It also suggests that there might be some therapeutic interactions between vasopressin and a form of psychotherapy called cognitive therapy. This is an area which requires exploration in future research.

The Possible Roles of Neurotransmitters and Receptors

Several of the participants of this symposium have implied that the catecholamine hypothesis is dead. If by that it is meant that the level of neurotransmitter (low in depression and elevated in mania) is no longer considered the *primary* determinant of affective state, I would agree. But it should by no means imply that neurotransmitters are no longer implicated as determinants of affective state.

I propose a modification of the catecholamine hypothesis which can be expressed by the following equation:

$$\text{neurotransmitter concentration} \times \text{receptor sensitivity} = K \qquad (1)$$

Equation 1, relating transmitters and receptors, while more comprehensive than the old and simple catecholamine hypothesis, is still greatly oversimplified. First, K should not be considered an absolute constant, but rather a value which probably must fall within a modulated range. Second, this equation deals with one neurotransmitter at a time when, in fact, there is substantial evidence that control of mood probably is based upon balances between various excitatory and inhibitory neurotransmitters. The nature of this interaction is not fully understood and the generation of an equation to describe their interaction, therefore, is not possible.

This is a tremendous oversimplification and will be discussed below. However, at least it brings the functional state of the receptor into the equation and implies that alterations in receptor sensitivity will be as important in determining mood as concentrations of neurotransmitters. This concept has several implications, not the least of which is that strategies for altering receptor sensitivity may work synergistically with strategies aimed at altering neurotransmitter concentrations. The use of triiodothyronine (T_3) suggested by *Prange* et al. [7] may illustrate this point. Tables I and II show that small quantities of this thyroid hormone, when added to therapy with tricyclics, cause a more rapid remission of depression in women, permit the use of lower doses of tricyclics, and convert many nonresponders to tricyclic antidepressant therapy into responders. This treatment is commonly employed in Europe and Japan but not in the United States. One reason for its lack of use in this country probably reflects, in large measure, the dominance of the early catecholamine hypothesis which focused so exclusively on neurotransmitter concentration.

Why do very small doses of thyroid hormone interact therapeutically with tricyclic antidepressants? We cannot be entirely sure. The rationale for using thyroid hormone in the study of *Prange* et al. [7] was based on a consideration of the role of this hormone in the functioning of catecholamines in the peripheral tissues of animals. The hypothyroid rat is sluggish, has lowered body temperature, low blood pressure, bradycardia, and appears as if seriously deficient in catecholamines. In fact, studies of peripheral catecholamine levels and turnover show that catecholamines are substantially higher than normal [8].

The hyperthyroid animal, on the other hand, is very active, has a high metabolic rate, tachycardia, and hypertension, suggesting high catecholamine levels. In fact, catecholamine levels are low [9]. A plausible explanation for these paradoxic findings is that thyroid hormone alters the sensitivity of the peripheral receptors, or of the receptor-effector complexes, in a fashion that permits a given concentration of catecholamines to be more effective. This was the reason for employing T_3 along with imipramine in the study described. Clinically, this approach works even though there is no unequivocal evidence that central norepinephrine (NE) receptors are reduced in hypothyroidism. Central dopamine receptors recently have been shown to be reduced in hypothyroidism [10].

The early work of *Cannon and Rosenbleuth* [11] showed that the receptor is capable of change in sensitivity. These workers demonstrated that receptors are adaptive structures whose sensitivity increases markedly when their neurotransmitter input is eliminated by surgical denervation of the presynaptic neuron. The experimental manipulation of receptor sensitivity, in the interest of clinical therapeutics, is still in its infancy. *Friedhoff* [12] has obtained some interesting preliminary responses to the pharmacologic manipulation of dopamine receptor sensitivity by flooding with levodopa, and then rapidly withdrawing this amine in patients with schizophrenia, tardive dyskinesia, and Gilles de la Tourette syndrome.

Although not directly relevant to psychiatry, it has been shown that the number of insulin receptors on monocytes from diabetes can be increased, and hence rendered more effective, by exercise. Thus, at rest, specific binding of insulin to monocytes is 69% higher in athletes than in sedentary controls [13].

Contrarily, the monocytes of obese patients bind less insulin than the monocytes of normal subjects. In obese patients, the concentration of insulin receptors per monocyte is approximately 50% of the normal value [14]. Exer-

Table 1. Thyroid hormones in combination with tricyclics in untreated depressed patients [41]

Authors	Dose[1]	Patients	n	Blind	Control	Type	Results and comment
Prange et al. (1969)	150 mg IMI q.d., 25 μg T_3 q.d. or P, days 4–28	women with primary depression, mostly unipolar; motor retardation	20	double	placebo against T_3	parallel comparison	T_3-treated patients achieved remission twice as fast as controls
Wilson et al. (1970)	150 mg IMI q.d., 25 μg T_3 q.d. or P, days 4–28	women with primary depression, mostly unipolar; no motor retardation; some agitated	20	double	placebo against T_3	parallel comparison	T_3-treated patients achieved remission twice as fast as controls
Prange (1971)	150 mg IMI q.d., 25 μg T_3 q.d. or P, days 4–28	men with primary depression, mostly unipolar; mixed retarded and non-retarded	10	double	placebo against T_3	parallel comparison	no T_3 advantage; patients showed a prompter IMI response than women in preceding studies
Feighner et al. (1972)	200 mg IMI q.d., 25 μg T_3 q.d. or P, days 2–11	consecutive patients with primary depression	49	double	placebo against T_3	parallel comparison	nonsignificant trend for T_3-treated patients to improve more rapidly than control patients

Wheatley (1972)	100 mg AMI q.d., 20 or 40 μg T₃ q.d., or P, days 4–28	men and women; depressed outpatients	57	double placebo against T₃	parallel comparisons	both doses of T₃ were significantly more effective than P; larger dose of T₃ tended to be more effective; women profited more from T₃ than men
Coppen et al. (1972)	150 mg IMI q.d., 25 μg T₃ q.d. or P, days 1–14; or 9 g L-tryptophan q.d., 25 μg T₃ q.d. or P, days 1–14	men and women with severe unipolar depression	30	double placebo against T₃	parallel comparison	T₃ potentiated response to IMI but not to L-tryptophan; T₃ effect limited to women, all of whom achieved depression scores of 0
Steiner et al. (1978)	150 mg IMI q.d., 25 g T₃ or P, days 1–35 or ECT alone	women with endogenous depression, unipolar or bipolar	12	double placebo against T₃	parallel comparison	all treatments equally effective, 3 of 4 patients being "responders" in each group

¹IMI = Imipramine; T₃ = triiodothyronine; AMI = amitriptyline; P = placebo.

(Reprinted by permission from A. Dunn and C.B. Nemeroff, (eds.): "Hormones of the thyroid axis and behavior," in *Behavioral Neuroendocrinology*, Chapter 13, Table 6 and Table 7. Copyright 1981, Spectrum Publications, Inc., New York.)

Table II. Thyroid hormones in combination with tricyclics in depressed patients who did not respond to tricyclics alone [41]

Authors	Dose[1]	Patients	n	Blind	Control	Type	Comment
Earle (1970)	IMI, AMI and protrypt in various doses, 25 μg T_3	men and women with retarded depression	25	single	none	before–after comparison	70% showed improvement under T_3 and tricyclics
Ogura et al. (1974)	various tricyclics, 20–30 μg T_3	men and women, old and young, unipolar and bipolar depressed	44	single	none	before–after comparison	66% showed a good to excellent response after T_3 was added, usually within 4 days
Caralca et al. (1974)	various doses of AMI or chlor-IMI; various doses of T_1-T_3 preparation	men and women, depressed patients, 42–52 years old	16	single	none	before–after comparison	thyroid preparations effective, especially with chlor-IMI
Banki (1975)	75–200 mg AMI q.d., 100–300 mg tri-IMI q.d., 20–40 μg T_3 after day 10	men and women, hospitalized depressed patients, all of whom had shown a poor TCA response after 10 days	96	single	increased dose of AMI to 300 mg of D	parallel comparison, after 10 days, between patient receiving increased tricyclic and patient receiving T_3	T_3 effective in 39 of 52 patients, additional tricyclic effective in 10 of 44 patients

Banki (1977)	75–200 AMI q.d., 20–40 μg T₃ q.d. after day 14	women with primary depression, unipolar and bipolar, all of whom had shown poor AMI response after 14 days	49	single	increased dose of AMI to 300 mg to D	parallel comparison, after 14 days, between patient receiving increased AMI and patient receiving T₃	T₃ effective in 23 of 33 patients; additional AMI effective in 4 of 16 patients
Tsutsui et al. (1979)	various doses of any of six TCAs; 10–25 μg T₃ q.d.	men with protracted primary depression who showed diminished TSH response to TRH challenge	11	single	none	before–after comparison	10 of 11 rated (globally) improved by T₃

[1] IMI = Imipramine; AMI = amitriptyline; T₃ = triiodothyronine.

(Reprinted by permission from A. Dunn and C.B. Nemeroff, (eds.): "Hormones of the thyroid axis and behavior," in *Behavioral Neuroendocrinology*, Chapter 13, Table 6 and Table 7. Copyright 1981, Spectrum Publications, Inc., New York.)

cise increases the number of insulin receptors per monocyte in such patients. This is also the case with adult-onset diabetics who apparently utilize insulin inefficiently because they have a low concentration of receptors. When these patients enter into jogging and other exercise programs, the number of their receptors apparently increases and their endogenous insulin is more efficiently utilized. Therefore, some patients may be able to discontinue completely the use of exogenous insulin. Could such physical fitness programs result in similar changes in neurotransmitter receptors? If this were the case, a physiologic basis for the reported effectiveness of jogging in the treatment of mild to moderate depressions might exist [15].

Whether aminergic receptor activity in depression is elevated, lowered, or unchanged is subject to controversy. A primary reason for this is that methods for the measurement of receptor sensitivity or receptor concentration are quite new and have not been adequately studied in affective disorders. Indirect evidence, based on NE infusion studies [16], showed that women demonstrated less pressor response to infused NE while depressed than they did after recovery from the depressed state, regardless of the nature of the treatment required to cause that change in state. This suggests that peripheral receptor activity is diminished in depression but, because NE does not penetrate the blood-brain barrier, it tells us nothing of central events. More direct evidence for diminished receptor sensitivity was inferred from the finding that clinical recovery following imipramine administration resulted in diminished MHPG excretion. Also, the addition of T_3 to imipramine increased the rate of recovery and caused a more rapid decrement in MHPG excretion [16].

Coppen and Ghose [17] conducted similar experiments and obtained data which led them to conclude that in patients with depression, the alpha-adrenergic receptors in the periphery show enhanced sensitivity which returns to normal with clinical recovery. The same patients showed no alteration in dopamine receptor sensitivity. *Bunney* et al. [18] suggested that the rapid shift from depression to mania in bipolar patients might be associated with the existence of a hypersensitive receptor in depression which becomes flooded with its neurotransmitter agonist during the onset of mania. Unfortunately, the authors offered no direct evidence for this view. *Friedman* [19] attempted to reconcile some of the conflicting literature by administering intravenous tyramine (a presynaptic adrenergic-releasing agent), NE (the natural synaptic transmitter), and phenylephrine (an alpha-adrenergic postsynaptic agonist) to depressed patients to determine whether they showed evidence of altered synaptic sensitivity. In his design, *Friedman* [19] measured the doses required for each of these agents to increase systolic blood pressure by 25 mm Hg. For all three pressor amines, the dose required to augment blood pressure by this amount was significantly lower among depressed patients than among controls. Therefore, he concluded that supersensitivity occurs in postsynaptic adrenergic receptors during depressive illness. Like all other investigators, *Friedman* [19] dealt exclusively with peripheral receptors.

Receptor sensitivity can be altered in two fashions. Alterations in the structure conformation of a receptor can alter the binding affinity of an agonist. This could lead to alterations in functional activity. *Pert and Snyder* [20] have suggested that lithium stabilizes receptors and prevents rapid shifts in their sensitivity by such conformational changes. Alternatively, shifts in receptor sensitivity may be due to alterations in receptor number per unit of surface. For many receptors studied, the latter mechanism seems more common in long-term adaptation. Whether central receptors are hypo- or hypersensitive in affective disorders remains a subject for research. Such research will not yield results rapidly because of the absence of animal models and the inaccessibility of the human brain for study. In considering future research, it is important to keep in mind that an absolute value of receptor sensitivity may not be important. Rather, that capacity of the receptor to show what *Prange* [personal commun.] has called "resiliency," that is, the capacity to show modulated variation in sensitivity, may be most important.

The Limitations of Pharmacologic Treatments

Pharmacotherapy has caused a revolutionary advance in the treatment of affective disorders. The use of lithium in the treatment and prevention of recurrent bipolar illness is the most successful treatment we now have in psychiatry. Its effectiveness may be compared with the use of insulin in diabetes. Lithium treatment can be used for many years and prevents devastating illness. While some undesirable side effects occur in some patients, these are generally minimal compared with the value of the treatment [21].

The benefits and risks of the modern use of electroconvulsive therapy (ECT) have recently been assessed by an APA Task Force [22] and, while there are some obvious disadvantages (e.g., amnesia and confusion), the benefits for selected populations seem to outweigh by far the risks. The speed of action and the percentage of patients with severe endogenous depression who respond favorably to ECT approaches 90%. ECT is, admittedly, aesthetically and conceptually unpleasant even when it is performed unilaterally. Nonetheless, it remains paradoxic that we reserve ECT for the sickest and the frailest patients, i.e., those who are actively suicidal and need rapid treatment, and those who because of age or impaired cardiac state cannot tolerate the tricyclics.

While our theories have evolved from the study of patients with primary severe affective disorder, we must not forget that the patients who visit psychiatrists and are treated for depression are a very heterogeneous group. They fall into what *Goodwin* [23] has called a "depressive spectrum" (fig. 1).

Many have depressions secondary to physical illness or to aging. A substantial number have chronic depression which seems to be characterologic. Most are nonpsychotic, unipolar, and acute depressives. For such patients, there is consensus that about 75% will show a symptomatic response to pharmacologic treatment, e.g., suicides, hospitalizations, alcohol and drug abuse, and work loss diminish. However, some tricyclic antidepressants have unpleasant anticholinergic side effects and significant risk of cardiotoxicity. Therefore, the more pertinent issue is how well do these patients feel and behave aside from their symptom reduction? This has not been adequately studied, but *Bothwell and Weissman* [24] reported on a 4-year follow-up of 40 depressed women who had been subjects in a research study of antidepressant medication and casework psychotherapy.

The symptom			The syndrome
Sadness	Normal	'Reactive'	'Endogenous'
Blues	Grief	'Neurotic'	'Psychotic'
Normal functioning Brief duration			Inability to function Prolonged duration
Symptoms of mood and cognition			Clusters of symptoms involving multiple systems including mood, cognition, sleep, activity, energy, appetite, and physiological function

Causative factors
| Environment | Biological predisposition / Genetic |

Treatment
| None | Psychotherapy | Drugs |

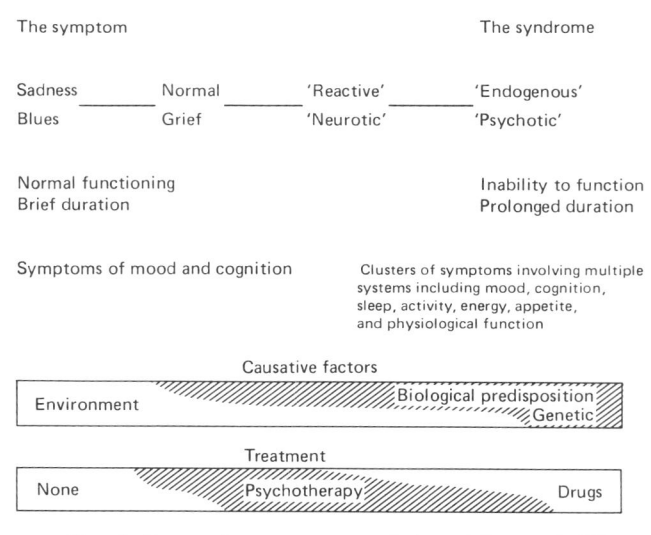

Fig. 1. Depression—a spectrum [adapted from ref. 23].
(Reprinted by permission from F.K. Goodwin: "Diagnosis of affective disorders," in M.E. Jarvis (ed).: *Psychopharmacology in the Practice of Medicine*, p. 222. New York: Appleton-Century-Crofts, 1977.)

In their depressed states, these women had typical depressive symptoms and were significantly impaired in their social judgment (as measured by work inside the home as a homemaker, or on an outside job, and in relationships with friends, extended families, spouses, and children). In their response to therapy, it was noted that improvement in social adjustment was slower than symptomatic improvement. Social improvement was the most rapid in the first 2 months of the acute episode, continued more slowly for the next 2 months, and afterwards was static for about 1 year. In general, the improvement was considerable, but it was not complete and did not reach the levels of their normal neighbors with whom they were compared. Four years later, 26% of the patients were as symptomatic as they had been when they first came for treatment. An additional 43% exhibited minimal or mild symptomatology not necessarily requiring treatment; 31% were symptom free. However, in terms of social adjustment, the large majority remained significantly impaired in the areas of work performance, interpersonal friction, and anxious rumination. Even in the group of patients who were symptom free, there was more impairment in interpersonal friction and in the marital role than was found in the control group.

These social and psychologic deficits apparently are treatable by psychologic interventions. Studies that meet the scientific standards for clinical trials and include randomized treatment control groups and independent assessment of outcome show that group therapy [25], marital/family therapy [26], or individual therapy enhanced the social functioning of depressed patients and resulted in improved interpersonal relations. These studies also have shown that psychologic approaches did not improve the symptoms of depression per se; they do not make depressed patients more energetic, nor do they improve appetite or sleep the way antidepressant drugs do. However, the psychologic treatments did improve social functioning. Together, the effects are additive (fig. 2). Patients who received both psychologic and antidepressant drug treatments simultaneously showed greater symptom reduction and better social adjustment [2].

Psychologic Considerations

The psychobiology of emotions, affect, and moods, and their role in survival of the individual and the species has been discussed elsewhere [27]. Briefly, subjective emotional states, expressed as affects and sustained over prolonged periods as moods in animals and man, serve in communications with

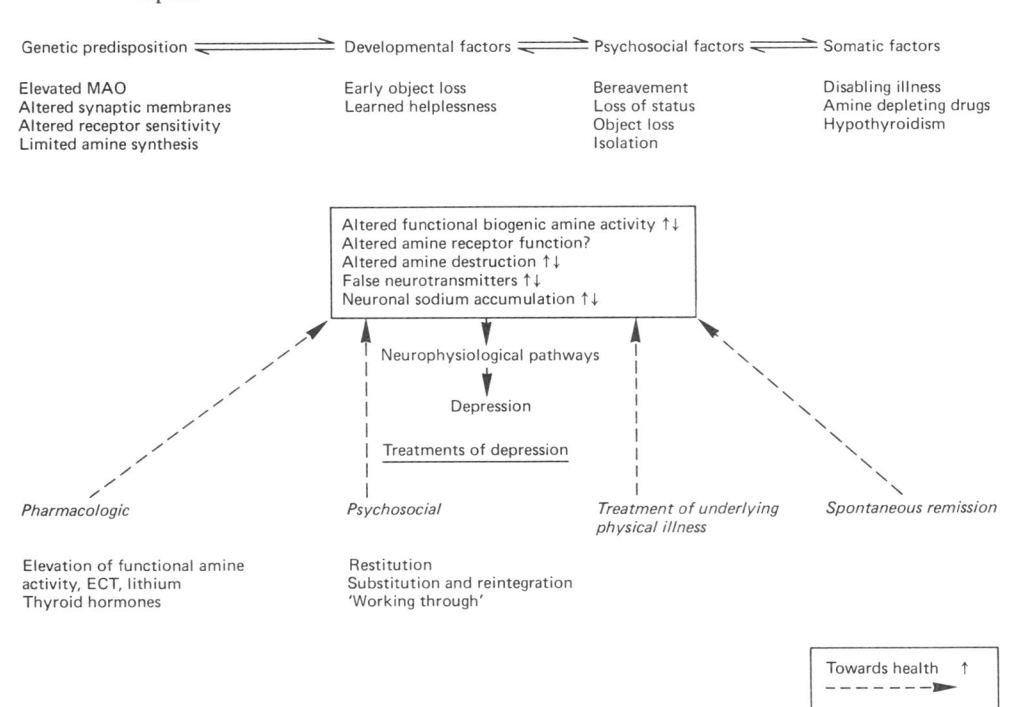

Fig. 2. A multivalent model of depression [adapted from ref. 40].
(Reprinted by permission from M.A. Lipton and C.B. Nemeroff: "The biology of aging and its role in depression," in G. Usdin and C.K. Hofling (eds.): *Aging: The Process and the People*, p. 49. New York: Brunner/Mazel, 1979.)

other individuals of the same or different species. The need to mate, to protect one's territory or one's offspring, to warn of danger, and to seek or to offer help may be communicated. The evolutionary significance of this to the individual and to the species is obvious. Emotions also serve to magnify and prolong reactions to environmental stimulation. Emotions interact with memory in the sense that emotionally laden experiences are more likely to be remembered than those which are not. The emotional experiences associated with hunger and thirst contribute strongly to consumatory or ingestive behavior. The expression of emotion in the very young is perhaps the most effective mechanism for communication of needs to the mother or to older members of the tribe or herd. Without such expression, the young and helpless would die and the species could not survive.

Every language has a very large vocabulary to describe emotions. Some of these express the same emotion along a continuum of intensity. Thus, annoyance, dislike, anger, and rage express the same emotion with different intensities and, presumably, have the same biology, with perturbations proportional to the intensity of the emotion. However, this has not been adequately studied. Other terms, like pity, shame, sympathy, and envy describe more complex affects. The biology of these feeling states is unknown. The work of *Schachter and Singer* [28] and *Schachter* [29] on the experimental production and manipulation of emotions suggests that there need not be a specific biology for each of the emotions. Rather, the same physiologic state may combine with different cognitive associations derived from the history and memories of the individual, plus the immediate environmental stimuli, to generate specific emotions. The fact that there is cognitive input into emotional states is pertinent to cognitive therapy, a form of psychotherapy which will be discussed later.

Emotions and their expression also may be looked at as psychologic equivalents of *Claude Bernard*'s principle of a constant internal milieu, or of *Walter Cannon*'s principle of homeostasis. There is in all living things a continuing attempt to maintain a constant internal environment, but it is often forgotten that this is never achieved except in death. The constant catabolism of life must be compensated for by anabolic reactions which follow after the ingestion of nutrients. Thus, there is constant fluctuation of pH, of blood sugar, of oxygen tension, and so forth within a well-modulated range. It is this modulation which offers the organism internal signals to eat, drink, rest, seek shelter, etc. If the perturbations did not occur at all, or were not recognized by the organism, there would be a constant catabolic decline ending in death. If, on the other hand, the perturbations were too large, the organism would swing like a pendulum between either acidosis and alkalosis or hypoglycemia and hyperglycemia. Complex chemical buffer systems and feedback reactions permit this careful modulation of the perturbations that are compatible with health. Similarly, the emotions represent the organism's psychologic response to the perturbations in both the external and internal environment. Failure to recognize them would not be compatible with life. Unbuffered overreactions to them also would not be compatible with life or, at least, with good health. Emotional disorders occur when these subjective feelings and their expression as affects achieve their own autonomy and persist inappropriately under changing environmental circumstances. For example, it is not difficult to find the circumstantial determinants of a first attack of mania or depression clinically, but later attacks seem spontaneous and without any detectable environmental precipitants [23, 30].

The many factors which influence the onset of depression or which, in an epidemiologic sense, contribute to the likelihood that it will occur have been discussed by *Akiskal and McKinney* [31] (fig. 2). It should be noted that, from an epidemiologic perspective, anything which increases the likelihood of the occurrence of an event may be considered a cause. From a clinical perspective, there is usually multivalent causality for the affective disorders. These include genetic predispositions, neurochemical alterations, endocrine changes, probably changes in receptor sensitivity, and environmental stressors. Whether environmental stressors have specificity in relation to mental illness is uncertain. Events which stress one individual may not stress another. Furthermore, there is no evidence that a particular stress is more likely to precipitate anxiety, schizophrenia, or depression. However, that undesirable life events precede the onset of depression seems well established. *Paykel* et al. [32] found that the number of such individual events in the 6 months before an episode of depression was three times higher in patients who became depressed, compared with a matched control sample from the same community. Furthermore, the types of events preceding depression tended to fall into the areas of marital difficulties, deaths, illnesses, and work changes. Even among bipolar patients, *Dunner* et al. [33] found that 50% of such patients had a stressful life event at the onset of their illness which could be related to its etiology. Difficulties at work, marital problems, and interpersonal conflicts ranked among the most frequent life events preceding illness and antedated first episodes of both mania and depression. The birth of a child produced depression but no mania in the first episode of bipolar illness. Subsequent episodes, however, did not seem to be associated with prominently recalled life events. Neither *Paykel* et al. [32] nor *Dunner* et al. [33] suggest that these events are a cause of depression. It therefore seems logical that restitution, substitution, reintegration, and "working through" such losses should contribute to recovery from depression. The various types of psychotherapy which are used in the treatment of depressed patients aim at increasing the patient's capacity to cope and adapt to these life stresses.

Psychologic Treatment of Depression

Until recently, the efficacy of psychotherapy alone in the treatment of depression was not supported by scientific evidence. Although over 200 publications dealt with the psychoanalysis and psychoanalytically oriented psychotherapy of depression between 1967 and 1974, *Lieberman* [34] found the data unconvincing because the studies were uncontrolled, lacked adequate numbers of subjects, and failed to employ criteria to insure that the patients were depressed rather than merely troubled. More recently, five types of psychotherapy—cognitive therapy, behavioral therapy, interpersonal therapy, group therapy, and marital therapy—have been tested in homogeneous samples of depressed patients using randomly assigned treatment in controlled clinical trials. These studies have been summarized and reviewed by *Weissman* [35]. Only cognitive therapy will be discussed here.

Cognitive therapy is based on the assumption that the affective response of depression is determined by the way an individual structures and perceives his experience cognitively. The depressed patient sees himself and the world negatively. Cognitive therapy differs from the more traditional psychotherapies insofar as the cognitive therapist actively engages the patient in the treatment process. Emphasis is placed upon teaching the patient to organize his behavior and to alter his cognitions about the stimuli he receives in the external world. Content of the therapy focuses on the here-and-now, with little attention paid to childhood material. The therapist makes no interpretations of unconscious factors, and a transference neurosis is avoided. Instead, if the patient has low self-esteem, he may be assigned a hierarchy of cognitive tasks and through the successful completion of these tasks can demonstrate the invalidity of his self-reproaches. Manuals on cognitive therapy of depression have been written by *Beck* [36] and *Beck* et al. [37], and the authors claim that the method is easily taught.

Cognitive therapy has been compared in clinical trials with behavior therapy, insight-oriented group therapy and, more pertinent for our discussion, therapy with imipramine. The study comparing cognitive therapy and imipramine [38] included unipolar depressed outpatients and a control group who were matched for age, severity of illness, previous drug therapy, hospitalizations, and suicidal ideation. The severity of the depressions is reflected in the subjects' average score of 22 on the Hamilton Scale for Depression. The authors claim that both imipramine and cognitive therapy were effective, but that 79% of the patients on cognitive therapy improved markedly compared with 25% of the tricyclic antidepressant-treated patients. Furthermore, more patients in the pharmacotherapy group dropped out. At 6 months' follow-up, 68% of the patients on drug therapy had reentered therapy while only 16% of the patients on cognitive therapy required such treatment.

What can be inferred from the results of this research about cognitive therapy? First, if one accepts the thesis that mood is a product of the interaction between a biologic state and a set of cognitions, as *Schachter and Singer* [28] demonstrated experimentally 15 years ago, it would follow that alterations in the patient's unique cognition of himself and his environment might indeed lead to alterations in his affective state. It is not yet certain whether *Beck*'s success can be replicated by other workers nor is it yet certain that his treatment will be effective in those severe depressions that are generally unresponsive to the environment, and that seem to be highly biologically loaded. But most depressed patients seen by the psychiatrist do not have pure endogenous depressions, nor are they psychotic. Because the patients in the study of *Rush* et al. [38] responded to antidepressants alone and to cognitive therapy alone, they may fit into the middle of the continuum of depressive disorders where they would be expected to be responsive to either form of therapy [23]. If this should be the case, then the combination of both treatments might be more effective than either alone. This has yet to be investigated.

Pharmacotherapy plus Psychologic Treatment

There was a period of more than 20 years when the concept of psychogenesis was dominant and psychotherapy was the treatment of choice. Then followed a period where the biologic factors contributing to vulnerability, to depression, and to use of pharmacotherapy were emphasized. The therapies for depression employed today seem to be based more upon ideologies than on the patient's needs. Psychologists and psychodynamically oriented psychiatrists use psychotherapy and neglect drugs. Nonpsychiatrist physicians and organically minded psychiatrists use drugs and neglect psychotherapy. Occasionally, this approach may work effectively if the biologic change occurs rapidly and the condition is detected early before the social and interpersonal maladjustments have occurred. But this is not usually the way patients present and it seems eminently reasonable that the two forms of treatment should generally be combined. For those patients who are so depressed that they are not environmentally responsive, ECT or pharmacotherapy as the initial step is mandatory; but after they have responded, some type of psychologic intervention might well be maintained. Even among outpatients, we find some who cannot tolerate pharmacotherapy and some who do not wish to enter into psychotherapy. Fortunately, for such patients, either treatment alone offers significant benefits. But for most patients, evidence has shown that the combination is superior to either treatment alone. In this regard, it is worth noting that *Parloff* [39] reports that there now exist about 140 types of psychotherapy. This is more than the number of drugs available for pharmacotherapy but, like the drugs, they can undoubtedly be grouped into significantly smaller numbers. Nonetheless, it seems likely that one of the major questions for the future will be how to select

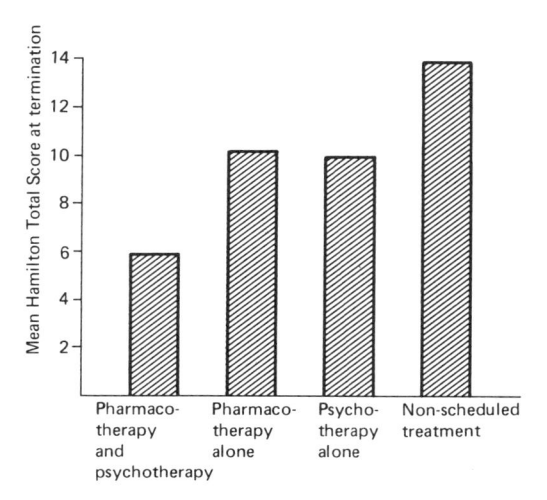

Fig. 3. Additive effect of pharmacotherapy and psychotherapy [adapted from ref. 2].
(Reprinted by permission from A. DiMascio et al.: "Differential symptom reduction by drugs and psychotherapy in acute depression," *Archives of General Psychiatry,* Vol. 36, p. 1453, Dec. 1979. Copyright 1979, American Medical Association.)

the right psychotherapy for a particular patient and how to combine it with the appropriate drug for that same patient. This will be a major responsibility of the modern psychiatrist (fig. 3).

References

1 Hartman, B.K.: Effect of tricyclic antipressants on cerebral capillary permeability: An action on a fundamental cerebral homeostatic mechanism. Symp. on The Psychobiology of Affective Disorders, Boca Raton, Fla. 1980.
2 DiMascio, A.; Weissman, M.M.; Prusoff, B.A.; et al.: Differential symptom reduction by drugs and psychotherapy in acute depression. Archs. gen. Psychiat. *36:* 1450–1456 (1979).
3 Hawkins, D.: Sleep and circadian rhythm disturbances in depressed patients. Symp. on The Psychobiology Affective Disorders, Boca Raton, Fla. 1980.
4 Vogel, G.W.; Vogel, F.; McAbee, R.S.; et al.: Improvement of depression by REM sleep deprivation. Archs. gen. Psychiat. *37:* 247–253 (1980).
5 Schilgen, B.; Tölle, R.: Partial sleep deprivation as therapy for depression. Archs. gen. Psychiat. *37:* 267–271 (1980).
6 Gold, P.W.; Weingartner, H.; Ballenger, J.C.; et al.: Effects of 1-desamino-8-arginine vasopressin on behaviour and cognition in primary affective disorder. Lancet *ii:* 992–994 (1979).

7 Prange, A.J., Jr.; Wilson, I.C.; Rabon, A.M.; et al.: Enhancement of imipramine antidepressant activity by thyroid hormone. Am. J. Psychiat. *126:* 457–469 (1969).
8 Lipton, M.A.; Prange, A.J., Jr.; Dairman, W.; et al.: Increased rate of norepinephrine biosynthesis in hypothyroid rats. Fed. Proc. Abstr. *27:* 399 (1968).
9 Prange, A.J., Jr.; Meek, J.L.; Lipton, M.A.: Catecholamines: diminished rate of synthesis in rat brain and heart after thyroxine pretreatment. Life Sci. *9:* 901–907 (1970).
10 Jahnke, G.; Nicholson, G.; Greeley, G.H.; Youngblood, W.W.; Prange, A.J., Jr.; Kizer, J.S.: Studies of the neural mechanisms by which hypothyroidism decreases prolactin secretion in the rat. Brain Res. (in press).
11 Cannon, W.B.; Rosenbleuth, A.: The supersensitivity of denervated structures; a law of denervation (Macmillan, New York 1949).
12 Friedhoff, A.J.: Receptor sensitivity modification (RSM) produced by chronic administration of psychotropic agents; in Fielding, Effland, New frontiers in psychotropic drug research, pp. 105–115 (Futura Publishing Co., Mount Kisco 1979).
13 Koivisto, V.A.; Soman, V.; Conrad, P.; et al.: Insulin binding to monocytes in trained athletes. J. clin. Invest. *64:* 1011–1015 (1979).
14 Bar, R.S.; Gorden, P.; Roth, J.; et al.: Fluctuations in the affinity and concentration of insulin receptors on circulating monocytes of obese patients. J. clin. Invest. *58:* 1123–1135 (1976).
15 Greist, J.H.; Klein, M.H.; Eischens, R.R.; et al.: Running as treatment for depression. Compreh. Psychiat. *20:* 41–54 (1979).
16 Prange, A.J., Jr.; McCurdy, R.L.; Cochrane, C.M.: The systolic blood pressure response of depressed patients to infused norepinephrine. J. psychiat. Res. *5:* 1–13 (1967).
17 Coppen, A.; Ghose, K.: Peripheral α-adrenoreceptor and central dopamine receptor activity in depressive patients. Psychopharmacology *59:* 171–177 (1978).
18 Bunney, W.E.; Post, R.M.; Andersen, A.E.; et al.: A neuronal receptor sensitivity mechanism in affective illness (a review of evidence). Commun. Psychopharm. *1:* 393–405 (1977).
19 Friedman, M.J.: Does receptor supersensitivity accompany depressive illness? Am. J. Psychiat. *135:* 107–109 (1978).
20 Pert, C.B.; Snyder, S.H.: Opiate receptor binding of agonists and antagonists affected differentially by sodium. Molec. Pharmacol. *10:* 868–879 (1974).
21 Shopsin, B.; Georgotas, A.; Kane, S.: Psychopharmacology of mania; in Shopsin, Manic illness, pp. 177–218 (Raven Press, New York 1979).
22 APA Task Force on Electroconvulsive Therapy: ECT: Report of the Task Force on Electroconvulsive Therapy, F.H. Frankel, chairperson (American Psychiatric Association, New York 1978).
23 Goodwin, F.K.: Diagnosis of affective disorders; in Jarvik, Psychopharmacology in the practice of medicine, pp. 219–228 (Appleton-Century-Crofts, New York 1977).
24 Bothwell, S.; Weissman, M.M.: Social impairments four years after an acute depressive episode. Am. J. Orthopsychiat. *47:* 231–237 (1977).

25 Covi, L.; Lipman, R.; Derogatis, L.; et al.: Drugs and group psychotherapy in neurotic depression. Am. J. Psychiat. *131:* 191–198 (1974).
26 Friedman, A.S.: Interaction of drug therapy with marital therapy in depressive patients. Archs. gen. Psychiat. *32:* 619–637 (1975).
27 Lipton, M.A.: Affective disorders: an overview of current concepts and ongoing research. Symp. on The Neural Basis of Behavior, sponsored by the Alfred I. DuPont Institute, June 1979.
28 Schachter, S.; Singer, J.: Cognitive, social, and psysiological determinants of emotional state. Psychol. Rev. *69:* 379–399 (1962).
29 Schachter, S.: The interaction of cognitive and physiological determinants of emotional state; in Berkowitz, Advances in experimental social psychology, vol. 1, pp. 49–80 (Academic Press, New York 1964).
30 Paykel, E.S.; Rowan, P.R.: Affective disorders; in Granville-Grossman, Recent advances in clinical psychiatry (Churchill Livingstone, New York 1979).
31 Akiskal, H.; McKinney, W.: Overview of recent research in depression. Archs. gen. Psychiat. *32:* 285–305 (1975).
32 Paykel, E.S.; Myers, J.K.; Dinelt, M.N.; et al.: Life events and depression: a controlled study. Archs. gen. Psychiat. *21:* 753–760 (1969).
33 Dunner, D.L.; Patrick, V.; Fieve, R.R.: Life events at the onset of bipolar affective illness. Am. J. Psychiat. *136:* 508–511 (1979).
34 Lieberman, M.: Survey and evaluation of the literature on verbal psychotherapy of depressive disorders (Clinical Research Branch, National Institute of Mental Health, March 7, 1975).
35 Weissman, M.M.: The psychological treatment of depression: evidence for the efficacy of psychotherapy alone, in comparison with, and in combination with pharmacotherapy. Archs. gen. Psychiat. *36:* 1261–1269 (1979).
36 Beck, A.: Cognitive therapy and the emotional disorders (International Universities Press, New York 1976).
37 Beck, A.T.; Rush, A.J.; Shaw, B.F.; et al.: Cognitive therapy of depression (Guilford Press, New York 1979).
38 Rush, A.J.; Beck, A.T.; Kovac, M.; et al.: Comparative efficacy of cognitive therapy and pharmacotherapy in the treatment of depressed outpatients. Cognitive Ther. Res. *1:* 17–37 (1977).
39 Parloff, M.B.: Shopping for the right therapy. Saturday Rev. *3:* 14 (1976).
40 Lipton, M.A.; Nemeroff, C.B.: The biology of aging and its role in depression; in Usdin, Hofling, Aging: the process and the people, p. 49 (Brunner/Mazel, New York 1979).
41 Loosen, P.T.; Prange, A.J., Jr.: Thyroid hormones and behavior; in Nemeroff, Dunn, Behavioral neuroendocrinology (Spectrum, Holliswood, N.Y., in press).

Discussion

Hawkins: Your analogy to diabetes is good, but I see a difference between this disease and depression. Once you get diabetes, you continue to have it.

This is true of many diseases that involve genetic factors. One question that comes to mind concerns the timing of the development of affective disorders in the life cycle. What does this mean in terms of the biology of the illness? Why do the severe, classic forms of depression, whether bipolar or endogenous, come and go? I don't know the answers, but it seems to make the analogy to diabetes less perfect.

Lipton: If you consider adult-onset diabetes, I think the analogy holds. An obese, adult-onset, insulin-deficient diabetic can lose weight, exercise and no longer be diabetic. The analogy, however, does have some limitations. For example, insulin lowers blood sugar in both diabetics and normal individuals. Antidepressant drugs, on the other hand, act differently in depressives and normal individuals. Normal individuals tend to experience feelings of dysphoria following antidepressant administration. Yet, when the same drug is given to the appropriate depressed patient, antidepressants produce positive feelings. Therefore, we are dealing with different substrates. Why depression is a self-limiting or a recurring disease no one knows. It is one of the questions that should be explored in future research.

Maas: I was very interested in your comments on drug therapy combined with psychotherapy. In my experience, the best results in the treatment of depression come from a combination of pharmacotherapy and some type of psychotherapy. I think it is absolutely necessary to give both.

Lipton: We would all agree that psychoanalytic therapy probably is inappropriate for depressed patients. However, behavior modification or cognitive therapy seems to benefit these patients. As Dr. *Maas* said, the best results may indeed come from using these types of therapies in conjunction with tricyclic antidepressants. But we must remember that only a few studies have been conducted so far and I don't think any definite conclusions can be drawn yet.

Secunda: I find that in first-case depression, about 50% of my patients respond within a few weeks to an appropriate drug-only treatment and need no further treatment after a few months. This figure is much higher than that generally seen. I think the reason for this is accurate diagnosis. We have to train clinicians to recognize depression accurately. Then we will be able to filter out that group of patients who are responsive to drug therapy alone and those who are psychologically depressed and need psychotherapy as well. The *Weissman* studies Dr. *Lipton* cited included chronically depressed patients and it seems natural that such patients would have social, cultural, and family problems associated with or created by a long-term illness. I think that is why such groups benefit from a multiple treatment approach. I do not think it would be necessary if depression were correctly diagnosed in its early stages.

Maas: Most of the patients I see are not patients who present with the first episode of depression. Perhaps this affects my experience with combined psychologic/pharmacologic therapy. Presumably, the first-time depressive can do quite well when placed on drug therapy alone and it is the chronic patient (who has lost his job, etc.) who benefits from a combined approach. Maybe we ought to look at this not in terms of pharmacotherapy versus psychotherapy, but in terms of length of illness.

Lipton: We must stress the need for precise diagnosis and early intervention in the treatment of depression. Both pharmacotherapy and psychotherapy are important in this treatment. I suspect that the optimum treatment will somehow involve selection of the correct psychoeducational program, whether cognitive or behavioral, *with* the correct drug which ultimately will benefit our patients.

Mendels: We all are aware of the heterogeneity of depression. Many studies use atypical populations, unlike the average patient we clinicians see in our practices. A large number of our patients who are clinically depressed respond to medication and become symptom free. The data from the Weissman study showed that a substantial number of patients had long-term symptoms and about 50% remained symptomatic after 1 year of treatment. Therefore, we must make a distinction. There are patients for whom drugs are highly specific and, provided they are given in a positive, supportive manner, the patients respond well. There are other patients who will require drug therapy along with psychotherapy to become symptom free. The point I want to make is that we must not generalize and take an either/or approach. Instead, we must define our patient groups more accurately.

Winokur: I think we need to focus our research efforts on the area of classification. We have reason to believe that there is more than one illness under the rubric of affective disorder. Until we know how many there are and what boundaries they encompass, our efforts in other research areas are hampered.

Katz: Classification is an important problem. I wonder whether so-called normal depressions (everyday "downs") are temporary phases brought on by changes in chemistry unrelated to daily life events. If so, when does this normal depression become an illness? Is it necessary to manifest physical signs of depression along with the experiential parts? Do you accept the notion of normal depression?

Winokur: I think there is a normal depression. It is bereavement. It is not related to heredity. It has all the symptoms of depression, improves on its own, and requires no treatment. On the other hand, a depressive *illness* involves a major change in the individual's life; the patient cannot carry on normal activities and feels different from his usual self. In these situations there is some reason to believe that psychologic factors may be relevant but they play only a minor role.

Mendels: We must be careful to distinguish between social and interpersonal consequences of depression and the illness itself. Also, when we consider drug therapy alone, we are not working in a vacuum. Of course we talk with the patient. We take a history and show a sense of interest, but in a nonspecific way, not in a directed type of psychotherapy.

Dunner: Psychopharmacology should involve a fair amount of psychologic support. I think we must identify that support, define its characteristics and teach clinicians how to use it. It is a very effective form of treatment which does not infantilize patients into expensive, long-term psychotherapy situations. Depressed patients who have social adjustment changes or psychologic changes must be well before they can enter into long-term psychotherapy.

Mendels: What about the importance of life stresses in connection with depression?

Dunner: These are difficult to study. Some occur before the onset of illness, others occur during the onset, and still others after the illness. They tend not to be discrete in time. Thus, some stresses which we assume to occur at one particular point in time actually occur over a longer period. It is possible that some people can discount these stresses psychologically. What might seem an overwhelming stress actually may be a minor stress experienced over time. Sudden life events probably have more impact, but in our studies they occurred randomly. Research on life events or life stresses should be carried out in collaborative psychologic or epidemiologic studies looking at possible important life stresses that may be involved in the recurrence of affective disorders.

The Psychobiology of Affective Disorders. Pfizer Symp. Depression, Boca Raton 1980, pp. 201–207 (Karger, Basel 1980)

Summary of New Research Strategies in Affective Illness

Jay D. Amsterdam and Joseph Mendels, Editors

The papers presented in this volume describe a wide range of research efforts aimed at advancing our understanding of the psychobiology of affective disease. One of the limitations of a symposium of this type is that no matter how completely the authors present their material, there always remains new and important information which has not been fully covered. In this chapter, we will comment on some of the work covered in this volume and also note new areas of interest.

It is essential to emphasize our understanding that depression is a syndrome, composed of several distinct illnesses lying on a continuum from known etiologies (e.g., brain tumors, endocrinopathies) to those which are as yet idiopathic. Affective illness can be compared in many ways with the diagnosis of seizure disorder. The etiology of convulsive disorders runs the gamut from known causes to idiopathic epilepsy. Some seizure disorders appear to have a genetic transmission, others to be familial. Some types have an early onset (petit mal) and others a later onset (grand mal). Often, they are recurrent and may be complicated by a psychotic symptomatology. In many respects, affective disease is comparable to both conditions, being a heterogeneous group of illnesses with various factors contributing to its etiology and to its response to a special form of therapy. In this often confusing situation, it is important to remember that a particular finding, while not specifically related to the syndrome as a whole, may be important for a subgroup of patients.

Dunner reviews the case for distinguishing between unipolar and bipolar illness, summarizing pharmacologic, biologic, genetic, and epidemiologic studies to distinguish between them. It must be noted that these two conditions are not necessarily single, uniform clinical states. Unipolar illness may consist of several conditions (see *Winokur*'s comments on depressive spectrum disease), and bipolar illness may be separated into at least two states on the basis of differences in genetic, symptomatologic, and therapeutic response. *Maas* has presented data suggesting a biochemical heterogeneity of endogenous depression based on the biogenic amine hypothesis of affective illness: a norepinephrine-deficient and a serotonin-deficient illness. He also suggests that these two groups correlate with response to a specific treatment. The norepinephrine-deficient depressions respond to imipramine or desipramine, while patients with the serotonin-deficient depression respond better to amitriptyline [1]. This research strategy has been extended using the tricyclic chlorimipramine for the alleged serotonin-deficient illness and nortriptyline for the possible norepinephrine-deficient condition [2]. These claims must be viewed as preliminary and controversial. For example, the hypothesis is based in part on the claim that patients who respond to one class of drugs are nonresponders to others [3]. Before nonresponse can be reliably determined, plasma levels of the drug must be measured to ensure that the patient had received an optimal therapeutic dosage. This was not done in these studies. Another important strategy would be the simultaneous measurement of MHPG (the primary norepinephrine metabolite), and 5-HIAA (the serotonin metabolite) in the cerebrospinal fluid of a group of depressed patients and appropriate control subjects. If the hypothesis is correct, one should find a negative correlation between the two metabolites. Indications from current studies are that this does not occur. A somewhat different approach has emphasized possible differences in norepinephrine metabolism of unipolar and bipolar patients, with MHPG levels being lower in the bipolar patients [4]. In our judgment, it would not be practical for general psychiatrists to determine 24-hour urinary MHPG levels, or CSF 5-HIAA levels, in their patients as a predictor of treatment response.

Most antidepressant drugs affect aspects of serotonin function as well as norepinephrine metabolism, and the indolealkylamine system may also be involved in the psychobiology of depression. Recent studies by *Savage* et al. [5] are beginning to throw some light on the possible functional alterations in this system with antidepressant treatments. The evidence of a possible involvement of the serotonin system in the development of depression was reviewed in detail (see chapter by *Amsterdam and Mendels*).

In an extension of the biogenic amine theory of depression, recent research has focused on possible alterations in the sensitivity of amine receptors on CNS nerve cells. An interesting model for alterations in receptor sensitivity is found in the pineal gland, which displays daily or circadian changes in cell receptor sensitivity.

Frazer, in his discussion, throws some light on the interrelationship between pineal function, neurotransmitter, and cell receptor sensitivity in depression. He describes how the sensitivity of noradrenergic receptors is altered by chronic exposure to antidepressant drugs. This finding has important implications for our understanding of the mechanism of drug action. It may ultimately throw some light on the pathogenesis of depression, and the reason why hormone release is often abnormal in some depressed patients. Cells which contain hormones, located in the hypothalamus, pituitary, and pineal glands, also have specific cell membrane receptors which seem to be influenced by neurotransmitters. Possible alterations in the sensitivity of these receptors might be one cause for the abnormal neuroendocrine findings in depression.

While the catecholamine and indolamine theories have occupied much of our attention, it is possible that other neurotransmitter systems may be involved in the biology of depression. Attention was focused on norepinephrine and serotonin and their metabolites, because the methodologies for measuring them were developed ahead of those for other neurotransmitter systems. Investigators are now beginning to focus on gamma-aminobutyric acid (GABA), dopamine, histamine, and cholinergic systems in the CNS.

Janowsky suggests a role for cholinergic mechanisms in the regulation of mood and possibly in the etiology of affective disorders. The cholinergic system functions in concert with other neurotransmitter systems, and drugs which alter central cholinergic activity may induce mood changes. For example, physostigmine has been found to have antimanic effects in some hypomanic and manic patients. Additionally, many tricyclic antidepressants possess significant anticholinergic properties which may be involved in their antidepressant action.

Carroll summarized some of the current neuroendocrine studies in patients with affective disease, and stressed the potential usefulness of the dexamethasone suppression test (DST) in identifying a subgroup of patients with endogenomorphic (endogenous) depression. He notes that 43% of patients with endogenous depression and only 1% of comparison subjects had this abnormality in four separate studies. He suggests that the DST has a high predictive value for the diagnosis of endogenous-type depression, but recognizes that more than 50% of the patients with this type of depression have normal DST results. This abnormality may be owing to a dysinhibition of the hypothalamic-pituitary-adrenal (HPA) axis, which is under control of the limbic-hypothalamic neuronal network [6].

A variety of other neuroendocrine strategies are also being employed, and alterations in the hormone release of the hypothalamic-pituitary-thyroid (HPT) axis, hypothalamic-pituitary-gonadal (HPG) axis, and abnormal growth hormone (GH) response to insulin-tolerance testing (ITT) have been identified in some depressed patients. These functional alterations may represent either a change in central biogenic amine concentration at important nerve synapses or possibly an altered sensitivity state at the neuronal receptor site (see chapter by *Frazer*).

To date, the most consistent finding is a diminished thyrotropin (TSH) release after intravenous infusion of thyrotropin-releasing hormone (TRH) in approximately 25–50% of patients with endogenous depression [7–9]. *Kirkegaard* et al. [9] also reported that a persistently low TSH response to TRH after clinical improvement might predict an early relapse into depression. Other pituitary hormones (luteinizing and follicle-stimulating hormones [LH and FSH]) also appear to be abnormally released by TRH infusion into some depressed patients [10, 11].

Some depressed patients have a blunted growth hormone response to the insulin-tolerance test, indicating an impairment of the normal hypoglycemic response to insulin in these individuals [12]. Alterations in noradrenergic or serotonergic pathways in the CNS have been hypothesized to be responsible for this blunted response.

In addition to these findings, our group has recently identified some abnormalities in the hypothalamic-pituitary-gonadal axis after infusion of gonadotropin-releasing hormone (GnRH) with augmented follicle-stimulating hormone release in some depressed patients [unpublished data]. We have also noted blunted prolactin response after TRH [11] and insulin-tolerance testing in some depressed individuals. The significance of these findings is not clear.

While these neuroendocrine responses are intriguing, investigators have paid relatively little attention to the possible importance of an association between the perturbations in the various endocrine axes. Future research efforts in neuroendocrinology will probably examine whether an endocrine profile exists for certain patients with affective illness, and whether abnormalities in the various neuroendocrine axes are present in the same individual. The question arises whether these pituitary hormone findings are specific for depression or are epiphenomena, perhaps indicators of limbic system noise, as noted by *Carroll*.

Closely related to the neuroendocrine investigations are studies which explore changes in biologic rhythms in depressed patients. This research has focused on studies of sleep physiology, circadian rhythm alterations, and possible functional abnormalities in the β-adrenergic receptors on the cells of the pineal gland. *Hawkins* describes some of the more recent sleep EEG findings. Patterns of a shortened rapid eye movement (REM) latency and a diminished stage 4 (deep sleep) are present in many patients suffering primary (endogenous) depression. These sleep findings are now being used in a predictive fashion to identify subgroups of depressed patients, and to study associated treatment response [13].

More recent research efforts involve the study of pineal gland function and possible alterations in melatonin release from this gland during depression [14]. Melatonin is a neuromodulator hormone, synthesized and secreted in a circadian fashion almost exclusively by the pineal gland. Animal and human studies have shown that melatonin modulates release of both pituitary and peripheral hormones, regulates sexual drive and maturation, and is somehow involved in the regulation of mood [14]. Its synthesis is under the control of β-adrenergic receptors in the pineal gland which are normally activated by changes in environmental light. The rate of melatonin synthesis is partially dependent on the concentration of norepinephrine at the receptor and on the sensitivity of the receptor [15]. The possible disturbance in pineal gland function and melatonin secretion, and their relationship to the pathogenesis of depressive illness, are the subject of ongoing investigations.

Research in the mode of action of lithium remains very active. Lithium's role in the management of bipolar illness is now well established. Attention has been directed to the mechanism by which lithium crosses cell membranes and concentrates in cells, especially the red blood cells (RBCs) of depressed patients [16]. This is expressed as the ratio of the lithium in the RBC to lithium in the plasma (lithium ratio) [17]. The transport of lithium across the RBC membrane is mainly controlled by a sodium-dependent lithium countertransport system [16]. Some reports have suggested that the lithium ratio may be correlated with biopolar/unipolar status or possibly with therapeutic response to lithium treatment [16, 18]. There is some evidence that bipolar patients accumulate more lithium in the RBC than either unipolar patients or healthy controls [16]. While these findings are intriguing and indicate the possibility of a genetically determined alteration in cell membrane transport in some bipolar patients, the findings have yet to be confirmed.

Availability of new research techniques and methodologies has expanded the horizons of depression research. The development of sensitive and accurate radioimmunoassays for the measurement of brain peptides and tricyclic antidepressant drugs, radioreceptor binding techniques to identify and investigate specific membrane and intracellular receptors for drugs, neurotransmitters and hormones, and the development and application of gas chromatography and mass spectrometry have all contributed to an increasing ability to probe and understand the fundamental processes of affective illness. New and provocative studies which investigate possible alterations in brain hemispheric laterality and neuronal metabolism are currently under way. Clearly, there is an explosion of knowledge in the field of psychobiology of depression. Our task is to relate this knowledge to the clinical problem, to determine which changes are specific to depression, and to distinguish between alterations which may be primary or secondary to the illness.

Furthermore, many of the systems under investigation interact with each other and undergo spontaneous changes over time. There are constant efforts to maintain homeostasis by alterations in synthesis, degradation, or receptor sensitivity. An increased functional activity of one system may lead to changes in another. We must therefore avoid oversimplistic interpretations of complex phenomena.

Finally, there is the overhanging question of the relationship between possible etiologic internal events (genetic-biochemical) and external phenomena (life experiences). These interactions are of the utmost importance and must be incorporated into our formulations.

References

1   Maas, J.W.: Biogenic amines and depression. Biochemical and pharmacological separation of two types of depression. Archs. gen. Psychiat. *32:* 1357–1361 (1975).
2   Asberg, M.; Bertilsson, L.; Tuck, D.; Cronkolm, B.; Sjobvist, F.: Indoleamine metabolites in cerebrospinal fluid of depressed patients before and after treatment with nortriptyline. Clin. Pharmacol. Ther. *14:* 277–287 (1973).
3   Asberg, M.; Thoren, P.; Traksman, L.: Serotonin depression. A biochemical subgroup within the affective disorders? Science, N.Y. *191:* 478–480 (1976).
4   Beckmann, H.; St. Laurent, J.; Goodwin, F.K.: The effect of lithium on urinary MHPG in unipolar and bipolar depressed patients. Psychopharmacologia *43:* 277–288 (1975).
5   Savage, D.D.; Mendels, J.; Frazer, A.: Monoamine oxidase inhibitors and serotonin uptake inhibitors: differential effects on [^{3}H]-serotonin binding sites in rat brain. J. Pharmac. Exp. Ther. *212:* 259–263 (1979).
6   Carroll, B.J.; Curtis, G.S.; Mendels, J.: Neuroendocrine regulation in depression. I. Limbic system adrenocortical dysfunction. Archs. gen. Psychiat. *33:* 1039–1044 (1976).
7   Prange, A.J.; Wilson, I.C.; Hara, P.P.; Altop, L.B.; Breese, G.R.: Effects of thyrotropin-releasing hormone in depression. Lancet *ii:* 999–1002 (1972).
8   Kastin, A.J.; Ehrensing, R.H.; Schalch, D.S.; Andersen, M.S.: Improvement in mental depression with decreased thyrotropin response after administration of thyrotropin-releasing hormone. Lancet *ii:* 740–742 (1972).
9   Kirkegaard, C.; Bjørum, N.; Cohn, D.; Faber, J.; Lauridsen, U.B.; Nerup, J.: Studies on the influence of biogenic amines and psychoactive drugs on the prog-

nostic values of the TRH stimulation test in endogenous depression. Psychoneuroendocrinology 2: 131–136 (1977).
10 Brambilla, F.; Smeraldi, E.; Sacchetti, E.; Nagri, F.; Cocchi, D.; Muller, E.E.: Deranged anterior pituitary responsiveness to hypothalamic hormones in depressed patients. Archs. gen. Psychiat. 35: 1231–1238 (1978).
11 Amsterdam, J.D.; Winokur, A.; Mendels, J.; Synder, P.: Multiple hormonal response to TRH in depressed patients and normal controls. Conf. Int. Soc. Psychoneuroendocrinology, Park City, Utah 1979.
12 Sachar, E.J.; Finkelstein, J.; Hellman, L.: Growth hormone response in depressive illness. I. Response to insulin tolerance test. Archs. gen. Psychiat. 25: 263–269 (1971).
13 Kupfer, D.J.; Foster, F.G.; Coble, P.; McPartland, R.J.; Ulreck, R.F.: The application of EEG sleep for the differential diagnosis of affective disorders. Am. J. Psychiat. 135: 69–74 (1978).
14 Mullen, P.E.; Silman, R.E.: The pineal and psychiatry: a review. Psychol. Med. 7: 407–417 (1977).
15 Klein, D.C.: Circadian rhythms in the pineal gland; in Krieger, Endocrine rhythms, pp. 203–223 (Raven Press, New York 1979).
16 Frazer, A.; Mendels, J.; Brunswick, D.; London, J.; Pring, M.; Ramsey, T.A.; Rybakowski, J.: Erythrocyte concentrations of the lithium ion: clinical correlates and mechanisms of action. Am. J. Psychiat. 135: 1065–1069 (1978).
17 Ramsey, T.A.; Frazer, A.; Mendels, J.; Dyson, W.L.: The erythrocyte lithium-plasma lithium ratio in patients with primary affective disorder. Archs. gen. Psychiat. 36: 457–461 (1979).
18 Knoering, L. von; Oreland, L.; Perris, C.; Runeberg, S.: Lithium RBC/plasma ratio in subgroups of patients with affective disorders. Neuropsychobiology 2: 74–80 (1976).

Author Index

Akiskal, H.S. 15, 28, 192
Allers, G.L. 172
Amsterdam, J.D. 57–71, 201–207
Anath, J. 62
Angst, J. 14
Asberg, M. 63
Aserinsky, E. 147
Axelrod, J. 67
Ayd, F.J. 138

Baker, M. 20
Banerjee, S.P. 55, 80
Baum, T. 81
Beck, A.T. 130, 193
Beckman, H. 40
Bjørum, N. 171
Bloom, F.E. 80
Bothwell, S. 189
Bowers, M.B. 85
Broadhurst, A.D. 61
Brownstein, M. 80
Buchsbaum, M.S. 16
Bunney, W.E., Jr. 186
Burns, D.D. 61

Cannon, W.B. 181, 191
Carlsson, A. 80
Carroll, B.J. 9, 36, 38, 86, 88, 99–110, 163, 164, 165, 171, 175, 203, 204
Casey, D.E. 88, 89

Castrogiovanni, P. 131
Chouinard, G. 61
Clark, H.B. 111
Cobbin, D.M. 41
Coppen, A. 58, 186
Costa, E. 82
Crone, C. 116

Dahlstrom, A. 112
Davis, B.M. 94
Davis, J. 83
Davis, K.L. 86, 87, 88, 94
Deguchi, T. 80
Dengler, H.J. 80
Detre, T. 154
Diaz-Guerrero, R. 147
DiMascio, A. 178
Dunner, D.L. 10, 11–24, 28, 36, 37, 109, 163, 192, 200, 201

El-Yousef, M.K. 87

Feighner, J.P. 19, 151
Fieve, R.R. 11, 14
Foster, F.G. 153
Frazer, A. 37, 72–82, 132, 145, 164, 202, 204
Friedel, R.O. 134, 146
Friedhoff, A.J. 181
Friedman, M.J. 186, 187
Fugiwara, J. 62
Fuxe, K. 112

Garfinkel, P.E. 58
Gershon, E.S. 18, 25–39, 85, 176
Ghose, K. 186
Gibbs, D.M. 93
Glassman, A.H. 60, 138, 170
Gluckman, M.I. 56, 81
Gold, P.W. 16, 179
Goodwin, F.K. 40, 164, 188
Greenburg, L.H. 81
Grof, P. 131

Halberg, F. 157
Hamberger, A. 173
Hartman, B.K. 39, 111–129, 178
Hauri, P. 153, 154
Hawkins, D.R. 109, 110, 128, 129, 147–165, 175, 179, 197–198, 204
Hayes, J.R. 138
Henn, F.A. 173
Herrington, R.N. 62
Heydorn, W.E. 81
Hogarty, G. 6
Huey, L. 83

Janowsky, D.S. 24, 38, 39, 83–98, 145, 203
Jope, R.S. 95
Judd, L. 83

Author Index

Kakiuchi, S. 81
Kappers, J.A. 81
Katz, M.M. 1–10, 107–108, 175, 199
Kety, S.S. 25
Kirkegaard, C. 171, 204
Kleitman, N. 147
Klerman, G.L. 28
Kline, N.S. 134
Korf, J. 62
Krauthammer, C. 28
Kripke, D.R. 156, 157
Kupfer, D.J. 28, 88, 151, 153, 154, 165

Lefkowitz, R.J. 82
Leonhard, K. 11, 13, 26
Lieberman, M. 192
Liebowitz, M.R. 15
Lipton, M.H. 109, 129, 164, 177–200
Lloyd, K.G. 63

Maas, J.W. 10, 23–24, 37, 38, 39, 40–56, 98, 129, 145, 164, 176, 198, 199, 202
McKinney, W. 192
Mendels, J. 9, 24, 36, 38, 57–71, 72–82, 98, 108, 109–110, 128, 131, 145, 163, 165, 199, 200, 201–207
Mendelwicz, J. 25
Modestin, J.J. 86, 87
Moller, S.E. 61
Morris, J.B. 130
Moyer, J.A. 75

Muhkerjee, C. 81
Murphy, D.G. 41

Oppenheimer, G., 89
Otsuki, S. 62

Pandey, G.N. 30
Parker, D. 83
Parloff, M.B. 194
Paykel, E.S. 192
Perris, C. 14, 28
Pert, C.B. 187
Petty, F. 172
Pflug, B. 155
Potter, L. 81
Prange, A.J., Jr. 180, 181, 187
Preskorn, S.H. 111

Raichle, M.E. 111
Rainer, J.D. 25
Rall, T.W. 73
Raskind, M.A. 134
Renkin, E.M. 116
Risch, C. 83
Rosenbleuth, A. 181
Ross, S.B. 81
Rowntree, D.W. 85
Rush, A.J., 194

Sachar, E.J. 64, 160
Sarai, K. 81
Savage, D.D. 64
Schachter, S. 191, 193
Schildkraut, J.J. 40
Schlesser, M.A. 171
Schultz, J.E. 50
Schulz, H. 153
Secunda, S.K. 5, 108, 130–146, 198

Shaw, F.H. 85
Sherman, B.M. 172
Shopsin, B. 61, 86
Siggins, G.R. 50
Singer, J. 191, 193
Sitarm, N. 88, 89
Snyder, F. 153
Snyder, S.H. 187
Sporn, J.R. 82
Sulser, F. 74
Sutherland, E.W. 73
Swanson, L.W. 111

Tamminga, C. 88
Taylor, A. 82
Thesleff, S. 82
Tolle, R. 155
Trendelenburg, U. 82

VanKammen, D.P. 41
VanPraag, H.M. 62, 63
VanValkenburg, C. 28
Vetulani, J. 74
Vogel, F. 161
Vogel, G.W. 154, 155

Wehr, T.A. 158, 159
Weiss, B. 82
Weissman, M.M. 189, 193
Weitzman, E.G. 156
Williams, L.T. 81
Wilson, R. 182
Winokur, G.A. 14, 37, 145, 166–176, 199–200, 201
Wolfe, B.B. 82

Yung Huang 40–56

Subject Index

Acetylcholine
  effects on, cortisol 92–94
  neurohormone regulation 93
ACTH. See adrenocorticotropic hormone
Activation-Inhibition (A-I) Scale 90
Adrenergic receptors 72–82
  activation of 72–73
  and adenylate cyclase 75
  and cyclic adenosine 3',5-monophosphate (cAMP) 73
  and catecholamines 73
  and desmethylimipramine (DMI) 73–76
  and imipramine 73
  and saline 73
  beta 78
    effect of norepinephrine on 73
  binding studies 77–80
Adrenocorticotropic hormone (ACTH) 100–103
  secretion of 101
Affective disorders
  biogenetics of
    genetic markers 29–30
  and dexamethasone suppression test (DST) 102–110
  and family incidence of alcoholism
    cyclothymic personality 15, 29
    schizoaffective disorders 170–171
    suicide 13–14, 63–64
  and 3-methoxy-4-hydroxyphenylglycol (MHPG) 17, 47–48, 176, 178
    urinary excretion of
  and probenecid technique 60
  and serotonin 57–71
    deficiency of
  and thyroid stimulating hormone (TSH) 16, 65, 171
  and thyrotropin releasing hormone (TRH) 16, 65, 171
  bipolar illness
    bipolar I 14
    bipolar II 14
    genetic transmission of 17–18
    "masked depression" 5
    and postpartum depression 59, 167
    and suicide 13–14
      family incidence of 14
    treatment of, with electroconvulsive therapy (ECT) 7, 169, 187
  DSM-III evaluation 19
  United States-United Kingdom study of 4–5
Allopurinal 61
Alpha adrenergic antagonist 186
Alphamethylparatyrosine 178
Amine
  measurement of metabolites 60–61
Amitriptyline
  differential symptom reduction with 178–179
  effect on sleep disturbance 178–179
Amphetamines
  response to 37–38
Anger Hostility Subscale 91

Subject Index

Antiadrenergic drugs 84–85
  reserpine 84
Anticholinergic activity 84–85
Antidepressants
  latency 73
Antidiuretic hormone (ADH) 117–118
Anxiety 11
Astrocytes 173
  receptors on 173
Astroglial cells 173
  alterations in 173
Atropine 93
Autoreceptors 43
  cell bodies 43
    and inhibition of impulse flow 43
  presynaptic 43
    α_2 receptors 43
    β receptors 43
    and neurotransmitter release 43
    and norepinephrine release 43

"Beat phenomenon" (see also sleep) 157
Beck Depression Inventory 5, 90, 153
Behavioral therapy 172, 193
Beigel-Murphy Arousal-Activation Subscale 90
Beigel-Murphy Mania Rating Scale 90
Beigel-Murphy Total Mania Scale 90
Biogenetics 18
Bipolar depression (see also under depression)
  bipolar I 14
  bipolar II 14
  bipolar-like disorders
    non-genetic mania 28
  Dexamethasone Suppression Test (DST) for 104
  and electroconvulsive therapy (ECT) 169, 187
  genetic transmission of 25–26
  and "masked depression" 5
  and suicidal behavior 13–14
Blood osmolarity 118
Blood brain barrier
  defined 114-115
  transport through 59
Blood pressure 83, 187

Brain
  auditory impulses 113
  cerebellum 113
  cerebral cortex 113
  hippocampus 113
  paraventricular nucleus 113
  pial vasculature 113

Cardiovascular system 135
Catecholamine hypothesis of depression
  and neurotransmitters 180
  and receptor sensitivity 180
Catecholamines
  reuptake by TCAs 120
Central adrenergic neuron system 112–114
  and cerebral capillary permeability 114
  physiological functions of 117–118
Central adrenergic vasoregulatory hypothesis
  and tricyclic antidepressants 118–119
Cerebral blood flow (CBF) 115
  alterations in 116
  effect of phentolamine on 117–118
  and net flux of water 117
Cerebral homeostasis 125
Cholinergic-blocking drugs
  atropine 88
Cholinergic nervous system 83–98
  in etiology of affective disorders 83
  and physostigmine 86–87
  in regulation of mood 83–84
  relation to other neurotransmitter systems 83
  and tricyclic antidepressants 84
Cholinesterase-inhibitors 85
Cholinomimetic drugs
  effects, in animals 84
    gnawing behavior 84
    and locomotion 84
  peripheral parasympathetic activity of 84
  reserpine 84
  and self-stimulation 84
  side effects of 84
Circadian rhythm 155–157
  biochemical aspects of 159–160
    and neurotransmitter metabolism 160
  in affective illness 160
  circadian arousal system 160

Subject Index

REM sleep latencies 160
SOREMPs 160
circadian oscillators 156, 163–164
"beat phenomenon" 156
and depression 160
environmental cues for 156
and lithium 157–158
light/dark cycle 156
Cognitive therapy 193–194
defined 193
and imipramine treatment, 193
use of cognitive associations 193
vs. biological basis for emotions 190–191
vs. homeostasis 191
vs. principle of constant internal milieu 191
Confusion-Bewilderment Subscale 91
Constant internal milieu, 191
Continuum theories 104, 194
Cortisol
ACTH secretion 100–103
and dexamethasone 102, 171
Cushing's disease 65
tests for
cortisol response 101
growth hormone response 101
Cyclic adenosine 3′,5-monophosphate (cAMP) 73–76
Cyclothymic disorder 15, 29

Delta wave sleep (see also sleep) 59, 152
Delusional thinking 167
Depression
and alcoholism 37
and antidepressants (see antidepressants and by drug)
Beck Depression Inventory
and schizophrenia 19
"beat phenomenon" 157
manic episodes 186
morbidity in 14, 18
response to lithium carbonate 12
diagnosis of 3–6
drug-induced
oral contraceptives 3
phenothiazines 3
reserpine 178

endogenous 171–172
in the elderly (see elderly patients)
epidemiology 191–192
eitologies 7
genetic 32–34
evaluations of (see evaluations)
follicle stimulating hormone (FSH) and 65
genetic factors
and mood disorders
bipolar 17–18
unipolar 17–18
in identical twins 25–26
geriatric patients (see elderly patients)
incidence of 1–3
and lithium 187
luteinizing hormone (LH) and 65
manic depressive disorders
postpartum 167–168
"masked depression" 5
measurement of
MHPG in 17, 176, 178
5 HIAA in 59–60, 172
National Institute of Mental Health Collaborative Study 4
neuroendocrine system and 99–100
pharmacotherapy (see also by drug) 194–195
postpartum 59, 167
psychoanalytic therapy 192–193
secondary 188
"stress induced" 10
treatment of
and orthostatic hypotension 138, 170
and suicide 13–14, 63–64
Type A 42
and MHPG 42
unipolar
"Depression Spectrum Disease" 29
and the dexamethasone suppression test 104, 171
genetic studies of 17–18
"Pure Depressive Disease" 14
response to lithium 17
treatment of
with cognitive therapy 193–194
vs. bipolar depression 11–12
vs. "everyday downs" 199

Subject Index

Depression-Dejection Subscale 91
Depression Spectrum Disease 29
Depression Subscale 91
Desimipramine 172
Desmethylimipramine (DMI) 75–80
  and activity of NE neuron-following cell complex 78
Dexamethasone
  suppression of cortisol 102, 171
Dexamethasone Suppression Test (DST)
  and Cushing's Disease 102
  diagnostic utility of 105, 109–110
  and "endogenous depression" 104, 105
  and glucocorticoid receptors 102
  and hypothalamic-pituitary adrenal function (HPA) 105–106
  and plasma cortisol levels 103
  and serum cortisol 171
  standard protocol for 103
  and thyroid stimulating hormone 16
  and thyrotropin releasing hormone 16
  and unipolar depressives 104, 171
Diabetes
  analogy to depression 197–198
  insulin receptors 181
  and exercise 181–186
L-dihydroxyphenylalanine
  administration of 12
Diisopropylfluorophosphonate (DFP) 85
  effect on manic-depressives 85
  effect on normal subjects 85
Diurnal rhythm (see also circadian rhythm)
  and secretion of 104
  and sleep (see also sleep)
Dopamine
  receptor sensitivity to 186
Dopamine-beta-hydroxylase (DBH), 113
Doxepin 130–146
  anticholinergic effects of 134
  antihistaminic properties of 133, 139–140
  and dibenzoxepin 134
  dosage 130
    oral plasma levels 134
  mechanism of action 134
  pharmacology 132–135
  sedative effect 139–140
    sedative-potential 141
  and sleep disturbances 140

DSM II 19
DSM III 19

Elderly patients
  depression in 138–139
  incidence of 136
  treatment of depression in (see also by drug)
    cardiotoxic effects of
      ECG changes 139
    and orthostatic hypotension 138
    use of tricyclic antidepressants 138–139
    and side effects 139
Electrocardiogram (ECG)
  QRS abnormalities in 136–137
Electroconvulsive therapy (ECT) 7, 187
  in endogenous depression 169, 187
  and suicidal patients 169
Emotions, 190–191
Endogenous depression (see also depression 171–172)
Erythrocyte catechol-O-methyltransferase (COMT) 11
Euphoria-Grandiosity Subscale 90
Evaluations
  Activation-Inhibition (A-I) Scale 90
  Anger-Hostility Subscale 91
  Beck Depression Inventory 5, 90, 153
  Beigel-Murphy Arousal-Activation Subscale 90
  Beigel-Murphy Mania Rating Scale 90
  Beigel-Murphy Total Mania Scale 90
  Confusion-Bewilderment Subscale 91
  Cortisol Response 91
  Depression-Dejection Subscale 91
  Depression Subscale 91
  Dexamethasone Suppression Test (DST) 16, 102–110, 171
    diagnostic utility of 105, 109–110
  DSM II 19
  DSM III 19
  Euphoria-Grandiosity Subscale 90
  Fatigue Subscale 91
  Feighner Criteria of Depression 19, 176
  Growth Hormone Response 91
  Hamilton Depression Rating Scale 90, 108, 193

Subject Index

Hamilton Depression Scale Retardation Factor 131
Hamilton Depression Scale Somatization/Anxiety Factor 131, 132
Insulin-Induced Hypoglycemia
Janowsky-Davis Activation Inhibition (A-I) Scale 90
Marke Nyman Temperament Scale 15
Maudsley Personality Inventory 15
Newcastle Index 108
NIMH Angeria Subscale 90
Profile of Mood States (POMS), 90, 132
  vigor 90
  elation 90
  friendliness 90
Research Diagnostic Criteria of Depression 4, 108, 175–176
Extraction fraction (E), 115

Fatigue Subscale 91
Feighner Criteria of Depression 19, 176
Follicle stimulating hormone (FSH), 65
Forebrain 123

Gamma-aminobutyric acid (GABA) 172, 173
Genes 25–39
  linkage 29
  markers 29–30
Genetic counseling 31–34
  empirical risk estimates 32–33
  and family history 32–34
  and psychotherapy 32–34
Genetic mania 28
Genetic markers 29–30
Genetic studies 20
Genetic transmission hypothesis 25–26
Geriatric patients (see elderly patients)
Gilles de la Tourette Syndrome 181
Glial cells 112
Group therapy 189
Growth hormone 91
Guanethidine 135–136

Hamilton Depression Rating Scale 90, 108, 193
Hamilton Depression Scale Retardation Factor 131

Hamilton Depression Scale Somatization/Anxiety Factor 131, 132
Helsinki University study of suicide 168–169
  and ECT 169
Hippocampal cells 50–53
  locus ceruleus responsive 50
Hippocampus 50, 99
His bundle
  electrocardiographic techniques of 137
Homeostasis 191
Hormones (see by name)
6-hydroxydopamine 121
5-hydroxy-3-indoleacetic acid (5-HIAA) 172
  in cerebrospinal fluid 59–60
5-hydroxytryptophan (5-HTP) 62–63
Hypermania, 86–87
Hypertension 5
Hypomania 28
Hypotension
  orthostatic 138, 170
Hypothalamus
  hypothalamic median eminence 99
  hypothalamic-pituitary adrenal function (HPA) 65, 102, 104–105
  hypothalamic pituitary gonadal axis, 65
Hypothyroidism 181

Identical twins 25–26
Indole compounds 58–60
  measurement in, central nervous system (CNS) 59–60
  blood 58–59
  cerebrospinal fluid 59
  urine 58–59
Indolealkylamines 57
Insecticides (see cholinesterase inhibitors)
Insomnia 179
Iprindole 50–51
  effect on NE neuron-following cell complex 50–51
  and firing rates of LC-responsive hippocampal cells 50

Janowsky-Davis Activation Inhibition (A-I) Scale 90

Subject Index

"Learned helplessness" model 172
Left bundle branch block 135
Limbic forebrain 111
Limbic system
  "noise" 106, 107
Lithium 94–95
  prophylactic use of 187
    in bipolar illness 12, 17
    in postpartum manics 167–168
  transport system 18
Lithium carbonate (see lithium)
Locus ceruleus 112
  basal firing rates 118
Luteinizing hormone (LH) 65

Manic depression (see depression)
Manic episodes 86
Marijuana
  and physostigmine 87–88
  and atropine 88
  Δ 9-tetrahydrocannabinol 88
Marital therapy 189
Marke Nyman Temperament Scale 15
"Masked depression" 5
Maudsley Personality Inventory 15
Melatonin
  and central serotonin levels 66
Mesencephalon 57
Metanephrine 40
3-methoxy-4-hydroxymandelic acid (VMA) 46
3-methoxy-4-hydroxyphenylglycol
  (MHPG) 17, 176, 178
  and imipramine 40–41
  and tricyclic antidepressant therapy 47–48
    nonresponders 47–48
    responders 47–48
  excretion of 48
  in cerebral spinal fluid (CSF) 48
MHPG (see 3-methoxy-4-hydroxyphenylglycol)
Monoamine oxidase (MAO) 11, 30
Monoamine theory of depression 30, 99

Neuroendocrine "cascade" 99–100
Neuroendocrine regulation 99

Neurotransmitters
  mechanism of action of 106
Newcastle Index 108
Nicotinamide 61
NIMH Anergia Subscale 90
Non-genetic mania 28
Norepinephrine (NE) 40–56
  and autoreceptors 43
  degradation of 48
    and S-adenosyl-methionine 48
  and drugs
    desmethylimipramine (DMI) 40
    imipramine 41
  and postganglionic sympathetic fibers 75
  effect of chronic tricyclic antidepressant treatment on 41
  inactivation of 45
  infusion studies 186
  metabolism of 44
  NE neuronal systems
    modulatory inputs 45
  and pressor response 186
  reuptake of 45, 47, 121
    vs. blockade 45
  synthesis of 44, 47
    and tyrosine 44
    and tyrosine hydroxylase 44
    rate limiting step in 44
    regulation 44
  and urinary 3-methoxy-4-hydroxyphenyl-glycol excretion (MHPG) 40
Normetanephrine (NM) 40

Oldendorf technique 119
Oral contraceptives 3
Orthostatic hypotension 138, 170

Paraventricular nucleus 112
Parachlorophenylalanine (PCPA) 64, 178
Peripheral adrenergic (sympathetic) neuron system 112
  anatomical similarities to central adrenergic neuron system 112–114
Permeability
  capillary 114–117
    and blood brain barrier 114–115

measurement of
 and phentolamine 117
 and water 115–116
Pharmacotherapy (see also by drug) 194–195
 in conjunction with psychotherapy 10, 194–195
Phenothiazine 3
Phenoxybenzamine 121
Physostigmine
 and affective disorders 89–92
 cholinergic effects 86–87
  hyporesponsiveness 86
  overactivity 86–87
 effects on
  cortisol 92–94
  depressive symptoms 87
   antimanic effect 87
   induction of depressed mood 87
   inhibitory-anergic effect 87
  "inhibitory state" 86
 and marijuana 87–88
  effect on REM latency
 and lithium 94–95
 and other psychiatric disorders 89–92
Physostigmine salicylate (see physostigmine)
Pineal gland
 β-noradrenergic receptors 75
 biochemical responsiveness of
  to changes in light 75
 dark-induced alterations in
  in vitro 76
  in vivo 76
 innervations
  and adenylate cyclase 75
  and β-adrenergic receptors 75
  and isoproterenol 75
 and serotonin synthesis 57, 65–66
Placebo 38
Polysomnograms 153
POMS 90
 subscales 90
  vigor 90
  elation 90
  friendliness 90
Postganglionic sympathetic fibers 75

Postpartum depression 59, 167
 mania 28, 167
Postsynaptic receptors 45–47, 187
 and NE neuron-following cell complex 45
 and biochemical markers 45
 effect of drugs on 47
 sensitivity of 45–47
Presynaptic membrane 45
Presynaptic nerve endings 72
Presynaptic nerve terminals 72
Probenecid, 11–12
 and 5-hydroxy-3-indoleacetic acid (5-HIAA) 60
 and serotonin metabolism 60
Psychoanalytical therapy 192–193
Psychobiology of affective diseases 1–10
Psychogenic psychosis 194
Psychomotor retardation 15
Psychopharmacology (see also by drug) 172, 173
Psychotherapy 6–7
 in conjunction with pharmacotherapy 172, 173
Psychotropic drugs (see by drug)
"Pure Depressive Disease" 14

QRS abnormalities 136–137

Raphe nuclei 63
Rapid eye movement (REM) 147
Receptors
 dopamine 181
 in hypothyroidism 181
  sensitivity of 181
   and bipolar depression 186
   and lithium binding 187
    affinity 187
    resiliency 187
Research Diagnostic Criteria (RDC) 4, 108, 175–176
Reserpine 3
Right bundle branch block 135

SADS 4
Schizophrenia 170–171
Schneiderian symptoms 167

Subject Index

Scopolamine 94
"Secondary" depression 188-189
Sedative properties of drugs (see by drug)
Serotonergic system
  neurons 57
  receptors 64
Serotonin 57-71
  in affective illness
    in psychosis 66
    measurement of 5-HIAA 58-60
    relation to delta wave sleep 59
  antagonists 61
  and aromatic acid decarboxylase 57
  and auto-receptors 57
  biosynthesis of 57
    active transport in 57
    precursors 61-62
      and melatonin 57-58
    tryptophan-hydroxylase in 57
  and desynchronization of circadian rhythm 65-66
  and FSH 65
  and 5-hydroxyindoleacetic acid 58-59
  and 5-hydroxytryptophan 57
  indoleamine hypothesis
    and parachlorophenylalanine (PCPA) 64
    in animals 64
  and LH 65
  and mania 64
  and melatonin 57-58, 66
  and postmenopausal depression 65
  precursors of 61
  and probenecid 60
    and 5-HIAA levels 60
  and serotonergic neurons 57
  synthesis (see biosynthesis of)
Serotonergic receptors 64
  alterations in 64
  sensitivity 64
Serum osmolarity 117
  and water deprivation 117
  and water load 117
Sinequan (see doxepin)
Sleep 147-165
  abnormalities 147
  alpha waves 148

architecture 152
  and depression 152
  and shifts 152
beta waves 148
continuity 151-152
  and depression 151
and cortisol secretion 160
delta waves 152
deprivation therapy 155, 179
  and TCAs 165
  selective REM deprivation 155
  sleep phase advancement 165
disturbances in
  and doxepin therapy 140
early morning awakening 160
EEG activity 147
  distribution of 147
  K-complexes 147
  spindles 147
eye movements in 148
and improvement of depressive syndrome 160
insomnia 179
light/dark cycle 156
normal
  brain activity in 148
  heart rates in 148
  non-rapid eye movement (NREM) in
    distribution of 148
  respiratory rates in 148
  slow wave sleep (SWS) 148
  synchronized sleep (S-sleep) 148
NREM/REM sleep cycle 148
  abnormality in depressed patients 153
onset latency 151
oversleeping 152
phasic activity 153
rapid eye movement (REM) 150
  activated sleep 150
  activity during 150
    in the brain 150
    and locus ceruleus 150
    and metabolism 150
    and muscle tone 150
    in normal subjects 150
    and pons 150

Subject Index

in primary vs. secondary depression 150
and depression 150–151, 152–154
deprivation of 159
length of 150
  and circadian rhythm 156
  in depressed patients 160
  in normal subjects 160
  and sleep cycle oscillation 156
mean values of 151
phasic 153
"rebound effect" 153
shortened REM latency 153
  as a "psychological marker" 153
tonic 150
REM latency 153
  distribution of 153
sleep inversion 156–157
  and mood 157
  and performance 156
  and REM latency 156
  and sleep onset 156
  and wakefulness 156
sleep onset REM phases (SO-REMPs) 153, 160
  circadian rhythm 153
  during remission of depression 153
sleep patterns
  electroencephalographic/electro-oculographic (EEG-EOG) measurements
stages of 148–149
  state 1 148–149
  state 2 149
  stage 3 149
  stage 4 149
theta waves 148–149
and threshold for arousal 149
and urinary 3-methoxy-4-hydroxyphenylglycol excretion (MHPG) 159, 164
and use of electroencephalogram (EEG) 151
Zeitegebers 156
  and urinary free cortisol 158
  elimination of 158
  in a unipolar-depressed patient 158
Stress 192
Suicide 13–14
  and 5-HIAA concentrations 64
  and serotonergic function 63–64
Supraoptic nuclei 112
Systolic blood pressure 186–187

TCA (see tricyclic antidepressants)
Tardive dyskinesia 181
Tests (see evaluations)
Δ 9-tetrahydrocannabinol 88
Thyroid stimulating hormone (TSH) 16, 65, 171
Thyrotropin releasing hormone (TRH) 16, 65, 171
Tricyclic antidepressants (TCAs)
  amitriptyline 119–120, 122
  anticholinergic activity of 121
  and capillary permeability, 120
  cardiotoxicity of 135, 189
  doxepin (Sinequan) 122, 130–146
  effects on cardiovascular system
    in animal studies 135
    anticholinergic effects 121
    quinidine-like effects 135
  imipramine 122
  initial workup for use of 140–141
  iprindole 132
  mianserin 132
  and orthostatic hypotension 138, 170
  protriptyline 122
  side effects of 189
Triiodothyronine 180
  and tricyclics 180
  treatment of depression with 180–181
L-tryptophan
  and allopurinol 61
  concentration of plasma 61
  free plasma levels 57
  and MAOIs 62
  and nicotinamide 61
  and serotonin availability 57
  and tricyclic antidepressants 62

Tyramine 186
Tyrosine 44
  hydroxylase 44

Vanillylmandelic acid (VMA) 40
Vasopressin 179

and cognitive performance in depressed patients 179
and cognitive therapy 179–180

World Health Organization (WHO) 1–3, 4, 5